The Ultimate PALEO Autoimmune Protocol Cookbook for Beginners:

Easy, Nourishing, Anti-Inflammatory Meal Plan for Advanced Healing Based on the Latest 2025 Medical Discoveries

Victor Armstrong

Copyright © 2024 Victor Armstrong
All rights reserved.
ISBN:

The Ultimate Paleo Autoimmune Protocol Cookbook for Beginners
© Victor Armstrong 2024. All rights reserved.
Except for brief quotations included in critical reviews and specific other noncommercial uses allowed by copyright law, no part of this publication may be reproduced, distributed, or transmitted in any form or by any means, including photocopying, recording, or other electronic or mechanical methods, without the publisher's prior written permission. This book is protected by copyright and is registered with ProtectMyWork.com (https://www.protectmywork.com).

Unauthorized use, duplication, or distribution of this material is legally prohibited. The author and publisher disclaim any liability for any damages, injuries, or losses that may occur from using or misusing.

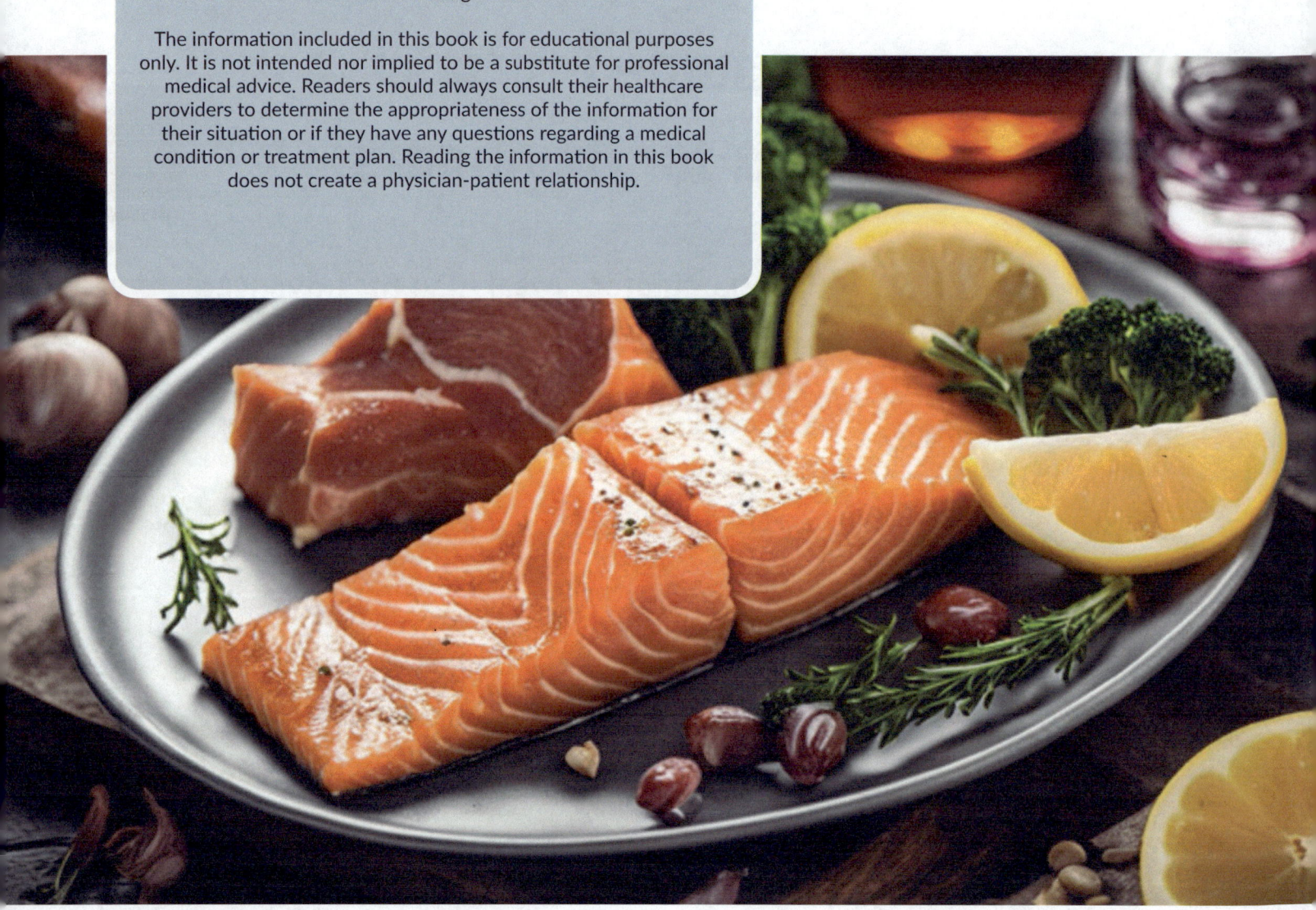

The information included in this book is for educational purposes only. It is not intended nor implied to be a substitute for professional medical advice. Readers should always consult their healthcare providers to determine the appropriateness of the information for their situation or if they have any questions regarding a medical condition or treatment plan. Reading the information in this book does not create a physician-patient relationship.

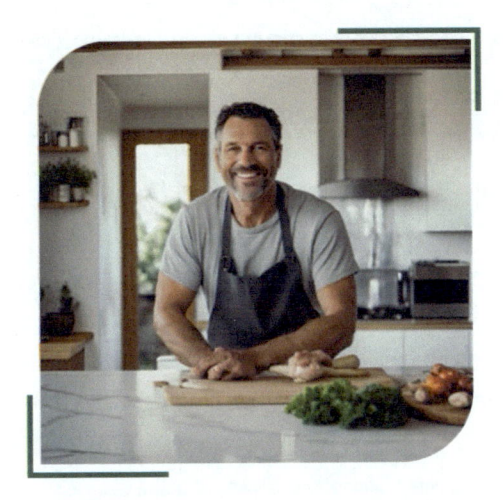

My Journey to Health: Healing Through Nutrition

I grew up in a small coastal town in Maine, surrounded by fresh seafood and farm-grown produce. From a young age, I was fascinated by the art of cooking. My grandmother, a talented home cook, taught me how to use simple ingredients to create flavorful, healthy dishes. As I grew older, my love for cooking deepened, but it wasn't until I faced health challenges that I truly realized the power of food as medicine.

In my early 30s, I was diagnosed with an autoimmune condition that left me feeling fatigued, inflamed, and unable to enjoy the active lifestyle I once loved. Traditional medications offered limited relief, so I turned to dietary changes. That's when I began my deep dive into therapeutic diets. I discovered the Paleo Autoimmune Protocol (AIP) diet, which focuses on reducing inflammation by eliminating certain foods, and I started crafting my own AIP-friendly meals.

As my health improved, I felt compelled to share my newfound knowledge with others. My first cookbook, Paleo Autoimmune Protocol Diet: A Beginner's Guide to the Autoimmune Protocol Diet, published in 2025, was the result of months of experimentation in my kitchen. Filled with nutrient-dense recipes, it provided easy-to-follow meal plans that helped countless people manage their autoimmune conditions while enjoying delicious food.

Inspired by the success of my first book, I didn't stop there. I recognized that people with various health needs struggled to find healthy and satisfying meals. My second book, "The Ultimate Low Carb Recipe Book: High Protein Meal Prep, Diabetic-Friendly Diet Cookbook with Easy Low Carb Recipes," also released in 2025, catered to those looking to manage diabetes, control blood sugar, or embrace a low-carb lifestyle. I focused on creating simple, high-protein dishes that made meal prep easy without sacrificing flavor.

My belief is that healthy food should be both accessible and enjoyable. Over time, I expanded my repertoire, releasing cookbooks that catered to other dietary needs, including keto and gluten-free diets. I became a trusted voice in the health and wellness community, known for creating recipes that are easy to prepare, full of flavor, and aligned with therapeutic diets. Helping others improve their health through food has been my passion, and it's been incredibly rewarding to see how my books have changed lives.

My journey, from someone seeking to heal myself to becoming a cookbook author and health advocate, is a testament to my belief in the transformative power of food. Today, my recipes continue to inspire people to take control of their health, one meal at a time.

TABLE OF CONTENTS

Summary Of Features And Benefits That The Paleo Autoimmune Protocol Diet Cookbook Offers: 6

CHAPTER 1: INTRODUCTION TO THE AUTOIMMUNE PROTOCOL (AIP) DIET 7
    1.1 Understanding Autoimmune Diseases 7
    1.2 Principles Of The Aip Diet 8
Main Reasons To Choose The Paleo Autoimmune Protocol Diet 8
Typical Top 10 Autoimmune Diseases 9
    1.3 Benefits Of The Aip Diet 10
Summary Of Benefits 11
    2.1 Inflammation And Autoimmunity 12
    2.2 Gut Health Connection 12

CHAPTER 2: THE SCIENCE BEHIND AIP 12
    2.3 Nutrient Density And Healing 13
    2.4 The Paleo Autoimmune Protocol (Aip) Pyramid ... 13
    3.1 Foods To Eliminate 14
    3.2 Foods To Enjoy 14

CHAPTER 3: GETTING STARTED WITH AIP 14
    3.3 Transition Strategies 15

CHAPTER 4: DELICIOUS AIP RECIPES 16
    4.1 Energizing Breakfasts 16
    4.2 Hearty Lunches And Dinners 16
    4.3 Snacks And Treats 17

CHAPTER 5: SUSTAINING AND PERSONALIZING YOUR AIP JOURNEY 19
    5.1 The Reintroduction Phase 19
    5.2 Lifestyle Factors 19
    5.3 Long-Term Success And Support 20
Frequently Asked Questions (F.a.q.) 21

CHAPTER 6: AIP BREAKFAST RECIPES 23
1. Green Gut-Healing Smoothie 23
2. Berry Coconut Breakfast Bowl 23
3. Tropical Detox Smoothie 24
4. Apple-Cinnamon Cauliflower Breakfast Bowl 24
5. Carrot Cake Smoothie 25
6. Creamy Avocado And Berry Breakfast Bowl 25
7. Sweet Potato And Kale Breakfast Hash 26
8. Plantain And Spinach Scramble 26
9. Aip Blueberry Coconut Smoothie 27
10. Baked Apple Cinnamon Breakfast Bowl 27
11. Carrot And Ginger Smoothie Bowl 28
12. Savory Cauliflower And Spinach Breakfast Bowl ... 28
13. Aip Sweet Potato Pancakes 29
14. Coconut Plantain Porridge 29
15. Zucchini Breakfast Hash With Ground Turkey 30
16. Aip Apple Cinnamon Smoothie 30
17. Collard Greens And Bacon Breakfast Wrap 31
18. Aip Pumpkin Breakfast Porridge 31
19. Aip Sweet Potato And Apple Hash 32
20. Butternut Squash And Sausage Breakfast Bake .. 32
21. Aip Banana Coconut Porridge 33
22. Aip Apple Cinnamon Breakfast Sausage 33
23. Chicken And Avocado Collard Wraps 34
24. Hearty Kale And Sweet Potato Salad With Ground Beef 34
25. Aip Salmon And Spinach Wrap 35
26. Gut-Healing Bone Broth Chicken Soup 35
27. Beef And Cauliflower Rice Stir-Fry 36
28. Herbed Turkey And Butternut Squash Salad 36
29. Ginger-Turmeric Chicken And Cabbage Soup ... 37
30. Lemon Herb Salmon With Asparagus 37
31. Sweet Potato And Beef Stew 38
32. Coconut-Crusted Chicken With Spinach Salad ... 38
33. Crispy Chicken And Roasted Vegetable Salad 39
34. Shrimp And Mango Lettuce Wraps 39
35. Beef And Spinach Stuffed Acorn Squash 40
36. Gut-Healing Turmeric Chicken Soup 40
37. Herb-Roasted Lamb And Root Vegetables 41
38. Cauliflower Rice And Ginger Chicken Bowl .. 41
39. Herb-Roasted Lamb And Root Vegetables 42
40. Seared Scallops With Garlic Spinach 42
41. Beef And Bok Choy Stir-Fry 43

42. Chicken And Artichoke Stew 43
43. Aip Turkey And Zucchini Skillet 44
44. Aip Salmon And Sweet Potato Salad 44

CHAPTER 7: AIP DINNER RECIPES 45
45. One-Pot Chicken And Vegetable Stew 45
46. Aip Shepherd's Pie With Cauliflower Mash 45
47. Roasted Garlic Herb Chicken With Root Vegetables 46
48. Aip Beef And Plantain Casserole 46
49. Moroccan-Style Lamb Tagine 47
50. Italian-Inspired Stuffed Bell Peppers (AIP Version) 47
51. Baked Cod With Lemon And Dill 48
52. One-Pot Beef And Cabbage Skillet 48
53. Aip Coconut Chicken Curry 49
54. Aip Beef And Broccoli Stir-Fry 49
55. Spaghetti Squash With Turkey Meatballs 50
56. Aip-Friendly Chicken Fajitas 50
57. Baked Salmon With Dill And Asparagus 51
58. Aip Braised Short Ribs With Garlic Cauliflower Mash 51
59. Ginger Sesame Chicken Stir-Fry 52
60. Aip-Friendly Chicken Fajitas 52
61. Pork Tenderloin With Apple And Sage 53
62. Aip Shrimp And Cauliflower Fried Rice 53
63. Roasted Duck With Orange Glaze 54
64. Greek-Style Chicken With Cauliflower Tabbouleh 54
65. Aip Garlic-Infused Chicken Thighs With Roasted Vegetables 55
66. Aip Beef And Butternut Squash 55

CHAPTER 8: AIP SNACKS AND SIDES RECIPESS 56
67. Gut-Healing Bone Broth 56
68. Turmeric Ginger Healing Tea 56
69. Kale Chips With Sea Salt 57
70. Sweet Potato Fries With Avocado Dip 57

71. Aip Plantain Chips 58
72. Zucchini Hummus 58
73. Cauliflower Rice Tabbouleh 59
74. Aip Salsa Verde 59
75. Crispy Brussels Sprouts With Lemon 60
76. Coconut-Date Energy Bites 60
77. Apple Cinnamon Chips 61
78. Carrot And Ginger Soup 61
79. Cucumber Dill Dip 62
80. Coconut-Lemon Energy Balls 62
81. Roasted Beet Chips 63
82. Aip Coconut Macaroons 63
83. Aip Baked Parsnip Fries 64
84. Aip Cucumber Avocado Salad 64

CHAPTER 9: AIP DESSERT AND BEVERAGE RECIPES. 65
85. Apple Cinnamon Baked Apples 65
86. Coconut Mango Sorbet 65
87. Blueberry Coconut Crumble 66
88. Pineapple Coconut Popsicles 66
89. Peach And Coconut Milk Ice Cream 67
90. Coconut Banana Pudding 67
91. Apple Ginger Tea 68
92. Berry Gelatin Cups 68
93. Aip Carob Pudding 69
94. Strawberry Coconut Milk Smoothie 69
95. Lemon Ginger Bone Broth 70
96. Coconut Berry Parfait 70
97. Apple Cinnamon Coconut Cookies 71
98. Ginger Pear Herbal Tea 71
99. Raspberry Coconut Milk Sorbet 72
100. Orange Cinnamon Hot Drink 72

4-Week Aip Meal Plan 73
Weekly Shopping List For The Aip Meal Plan 75
List Of Ingredients 78
About Me 79

SUMMARY OF FEATURES AND BENEFITS THAT THE PALEO AUTOIMMUNE PROTOCOL DIET COOKBOOK OFFERS:

Comprehensive AIP Guide	A detailed explanation of the Paleo Autoimmune Protocol, including fundamental principles, allowed foods, and phases.
Beginner-Friendly	Provides step-by-step guidance on starting the AIP, including elimination and reintroduction phases.
Nutrient-Dense Recipes	A wide variety of AIP-compliant recipes focus on nutrient-dense, anti-inflammatory ingredients.
Meal Planning	Offers meal plans, batch cooking tips, and shopping lists to help readers stay organized.
Reintroduction Guidance	Detailed steps for reintroducing foods after elimination to identify potential triggers.
Lifestyle Advice	Incorporates stress and sleep management tips to support overall healing.
Practical Cooking Tips	Advice on setting up an AIP-friendly kitchen, batch cooking, and meal prepping.
Diverse Recipe Categories	Categorized recipes for breakfast, lunch, dinner, snacks, and desserts.
AIP Pyramid and Visuals	It provides visual aids like the AIP food pyramid to help people understand food choices better.
Customizable for Other Diets	Offers suggestions for combining AIP with keto, low-FODMAP, and vegetarian/vegan diets.
Gut-Healing Foods	Focuses on gut-healing foods like bone broth and fermented vegetables.
Support for Social and Emotional Challenges	Tips for handling social situations, cravings, and staying motivated during the diet.
Frequently Asked Questions	A section addressing common AIP questions and managing autoimmune diseases.
Scientific Basis	Provides scientific backing on how the AIP diet supports immune regulation, inflammation control, and gut healing.

The Paleo Autoimmune Protocol Diet Cookbook offers a comprehensive, beginner-friendly guide to the AIP diet, featuring nutrient-dense recipes and practical meal-planning tips. It provides detailed reintroduction guidance, lifestyle advice, and support for social and emotional challenges, all backed by scientific research, making it a valuable resource for managing autoimmune conditions.

CHAPTER 1

Introduction to the Autoimmune Protocol (AIP) Diet

Autoimmune diseases affect millions of people worldwide, mistakenly causing the immune system to attack the body's own tissues. The Autoimmune Protocol (AIP) diet is a natural, holistic approach aimed at reducing inflammation and supporting the body's healing process. By eliminating certain foods and focusing on nutrient-dense choices, the AIP diet provides a unique method for managing autoimmune conditions that goes beyond conventional treatments. This chapter lays a foundational understanding of the AIP diet and how it can be used to effectively manage autoimmune disorders and improve overall well-being.

1.1 Understanding Autoimmune Diseases

Autoimmune diseases encompass a broad spectrum of conditions, including rheumatoid arthritis, lupus, multiple sclerosis, and inflammatory bowel disease. Despite their differences, all autoimmune conditions share a common factor: a malfunctioning immune system that mistakenly targets the body's own cells. In a healthy body, the immune system serves as a line of defense, protecting against harmful invaders such as bacteria, viruses, and other pathogens. However, in the case of autoimmune diseases, the immune system misidentifies the body's own tissues as foreign threats, leading to chronic inflammation and tissue damage.

There is no singular cause of autoimmune diseases. Instead, a combination of genetic predisposition, environmental factors, lifestyle choices, and diet contribute to this misguided immune response. Factors such as chronic stress, exposure to toxins, a lack of sleep, and poor dietary habits can all contribute to the development or exacerbation of autoimmune conditions. Understanding these root causes is crucial in developing a comprehensive approach to managing autoimmune disorders.

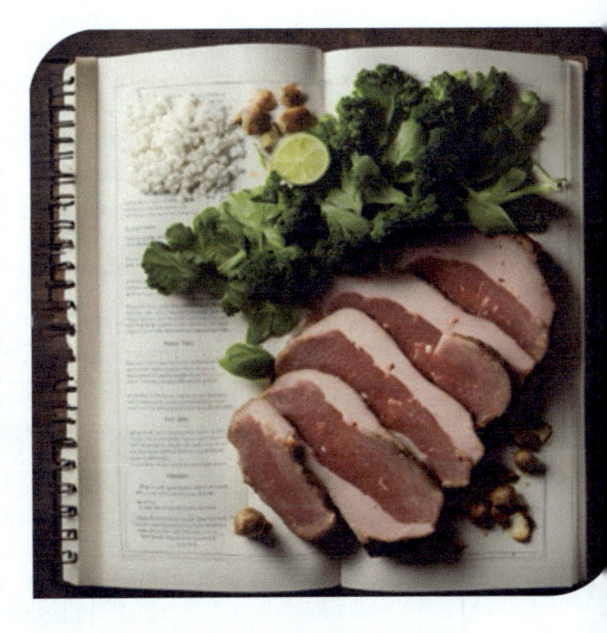

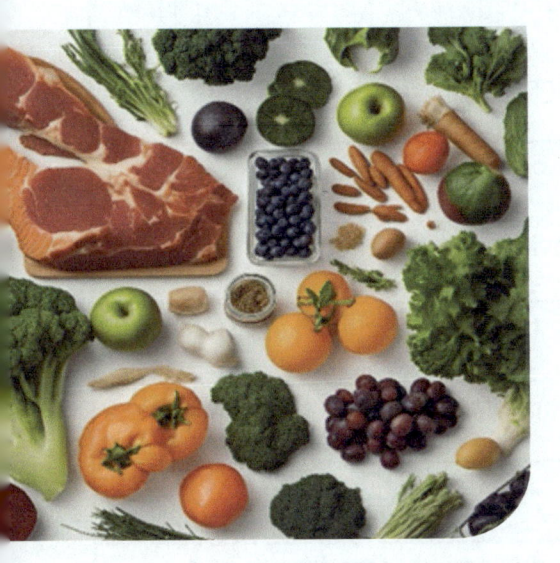

Chronic inflammation is the hallmark of autoimmune diseases. While acute inflammation is a natural, protective response designed to heal injuries or fight infections, chronic inflammation can become destructive, causing damage to tissues and organs over time. Standard medical treatments for autoimmune diseases often involve medications that suppress the immune system to reduce inflammation and provide symptom relief. Although these medications can be effective, they may also carry significant side effects and do not address the underlying causes of the disease.

This is where the Paleo Autoimmune Protocol (AIP) diet comes in—a natural dietary approach that aims to modulate the immune system, reduce inflammation, and promote healing from within. By removing foods that are known to trigger inflammation, such as gluten, dairy, grains, legumes, and processed foods, and instead focusing on nutrient-dense foods like vegetables, fruits, healthy fats, and quality proteins, the AIP diet helps create an environment where the body can heal. The AIP diet is not just about eliminating foods; it's about replacing them with nutrient-rich options that provide the vitamins and minerals needed for optimal immune function and tissue repair. The AIP diet empowers individuals with autoimmune conditions to take control of their health by addressing the root causes of their disease and supporting the body's natural ability to heal.

1.2 Principles of the AIP Diet

The Autoimmune Protocol (AIP) diet is a specialized extension of the Paleo diet, meticulously designed for individuals with autoimmune conditions. While the Paleo diet emphasizes whole, unprocessed foods similar to those consumed by early humans, the AIP diet eliminates additional foods that may trigger immune responses or contribute to gut inflammation. This targeted approach aims to reduce systemic inflammation, support gut healing, and alleviate autoimmune symptoms.

The diet consists of two main phases: the elimination phase and the reintroduction phase.

- Elimination Phase: In this initial phase, a wide range of potential dietary irritants are removed. These include grains (such as wheat, barley, and rice), legumes (beans, lentils, and peanuts), dairy products, nuts and seeds, nightshade vegetables (like tomatoes, potatoes, eggplants, and peppers), eggs, processed foods, refined sugars, and food additives. The goal is to reduce inflammation and give the body's immune system and gut lining an opportunity to heal. This phase typically lasts at least 30 days but can be extended based on individual needs and symptom improvement.

- Reintroduction Phase: After the elimination period, foods are gradually reintroduced one at a time in a systematic manner. This process involves consuming a small amount of a single food and monitoring the body for any adverse reactions over several days before introducing another. Reactions to watch for include digestive discomfort, joint pain, skin issues, or a return of autoimmune symptoms. This phase helps identify specific food sensitivities and intolerances, allowing individuals to tailor their diet to their unique needs and create a sustainable, personalized eating plan.

By focusing on these whole, unprocessed foods, the AIP diet ensures that the body receives the necessary nutrients to function optimally while minimizing potential dietary triggers. This approach aims to reduce inflammation and support overall health by promoting a balanced immune response and aiding gut healing.

Understanding and implementing the principles of the AIP diet can empower individuals with autoimmune conditions to take control of their health through informed dietary choices. By addressing specific dietary triggers and emphasizing nutrient-rich foods, the diet offers a proactive strategy for managing symptoms and improving quality of life.

MAIN REASONS TO CHOOSE THE PALEO AUTOIMMUNE PROTOCOL DIET

Reduces Chronic Inflammation	It effectively manages inflammation by focusing on anti-inflammatory foods like vegetables, fruits, and lean meats.
Heals Gut Lining	Eliminates foods that irritate the gut, promoting healing and reducing leaky gut symptoms.
Balances Immune Response	Supports immune regulation by eliminating common autoimmune triggers, leading to fewer flare-ups.
Identifies Food Sensitivities	The elimination process helps pinpoint foods that trigger autoimmune responses and discomfort.
Increases Nutrient Density	It focuses on nutrient-rich foods that provide essential vitamins, minerals, and antioxidants for healing.
Improves Energy Levels	Reduces energy-sapping inflammation and supports stable blood sugar through whole food choices.
Promotes Healthy Weight Loss	Encourages balanced, clean eating that supports healthy, gradual weight loss without deprivation.
Boosts Brain Function	Reduces brain fog and enhances mental clarity by eliminating inflammatory foods and toxins.
Supports Hormonal Balance	It helps regulate hormones naturally by reducing processed foods and toxins in the diet.

Minimizes Risk of Autoimmune Flare-ups	Decreases the frequency and intensity of autoimmune flare-ups by reducing inflammation triggers.
Lowers Risk of Chronic Illness	Reduces the risk of heart disease, diabetes, and other chronic illnesses through an anti-inflammatory diet.
Enhances Skin Health	Eliminates foods that can trigger skin issues, promoting clearer, healthier skin.
Promotes Better Sleep	Supports restful sleep by stabilizing blood sugar levels and reducing inflammation.
Encourages Mindful Eating	It helps develop a deeper connection to food, encouraging long-term, mindful eating habits.

TYPICAL TOP 10 AUTOIMMUNE DISEASES

Rheumatoid Arthritis (RA)	A chronic inflammatory disorder where the immune system attacks joint linings, causing pain, swelling, and potential joint deformities and erosion.
Lupus (Systemic Lupus Erythematosus - SLE)	An autoimmune disease causing widespread inflammation and tissue damage, affecting the skin, joints, kidneys, brain, and other organs.
Multiple Sclerosis (MS)	A condition where the immune system attacks the protective covering (myelin) of nerves, leading to communication issues between the brain and body.
Type 1 Diabetes	The immune system mistakenly destroys insulin-producing cells in the pancreas, leading to high blood sugar and requiring lifelong insulin management.
Hashimoto's Thyroiditis	The immune system attacks the thyroid gland, causing hypothyroidism, leading to fatigue, weight gain, and sensitivity to cold.
Graves' Disease	It is an autoimmune disorder where the immune system overstimulates the thyroid gland, causing hyperthyroidism with symptoms like anxiety, tremors, and weight loss.
Psoriasis	A skin condition where the immune system speeds up skin cell growth, leading to red, scaly patches on the skin that can be itchy and painful.
Inflammatory Bowel Disease (IBD)	Includes Crohn's disease and ulcerative colitis, where the immune system attacks the gastrointestinal tract, causing abdominal pain, diarrhea, and malnutrition.
Celiac Disease	An autoimmune reaction to gluten that damages the small intestine lining, causing digestive issues, nutrient malabsorption, and other systemic symptoms.
Ankylosing Spondylitis	A type of arthritis that primarily affects the spine, causing inflammation, pain, and stiffness, potentially leading to spinal fusion in severe cases.

This list explains each autoimmune disease, emphasizing how the immune system mistakenly targets the body's tissues.

1.3 Benefits of the AIP Diet

Reduction of Inflammation
The Autoimmune Protocol (AIP) diet is designed to reduce chronic inflammation, a fundamental factor in autoimmune conditions. By eliminating foods known to trigger inflammatory responses—such as grains, legumes, dairy, processed foods, and certain additives—the diet helps to calm the immune system. Inflammation is the body's natural response to injury or harmful stimuli, but when it becomes chronic, it can lead to tissue damage and exacerbate autoimmune symptoms. Chronic inflammation can affect various organs and systems, contributing to joint pain, skin rashes, fatigue, and even organ dysfunction, all common symptoms in autoimmune diseases.

The AIP diet focuses on nutrient-dense, anti-inflammatory foods like leafy greens, colorful vegetables, fatty fish rich in omega-3 fatty acids, and antioxidant-rich fruits. These foods help lower inflammation and provide essential vitamins and minerals that support immune regulation. Omega-3 fatty acids found in fatty fish like salmon and mackerel are particularly effective at reducing inflammation, as they inhibit the production of pro-inflammatory molecules called cytokines. This makes omega-3s a vital component in managing autoimmune diseases, often marked by elevated levels of inflammation.

In addition to omega-3 fatty acids, antioxidant-rich foods like berries, leafy greens, and cruciferous vegetables play a crucial role in reducing oxidative stress in the body. Oxidative stress, when free radicals outnumber antioxidants, can contribute to chronic inflammation and tissue damage. By consuming a diet rich in antioxidants, individuals on the AIP diet can help neutralize free radicals, thereby protecting their cells from further damage and reducing inflammation.

Healing the Gut and Improving Digestion
Gut health plays a critical role in immune function, and many autoimmune conditions are linked to increased intestinal permeability, often called "leaky gut." When the gut lining becomes compromised, undigested food particles, toxins, and pathogens can enter the bloodstream, triggering an immune response. Over time, this can contribute to systemic inflammation and exacerbate autoimmune symptoms.

The AIP diet aims to heal the gut lining by removing foods that may irritate the digestive tract and contribute to inflammation. Grains, legumes, and processed foods are often difficult to digest and can damage the intestinal lining. In contrast, certain food additives like emulsifiers and artificial sweeteners may disrupt the balance of gut bacteria. By eliminating these potential irritants, the AIP diet helps reduce stress on the digestive system and allows the gut lining to repair itself.

One of the critical components of the AIP diet for gut healing is the inclusion of gut-healing nutrients like collagen and gelatin, often derived from bone broth. Collagen is the most abundant protein in the body and is essential for maintaining the structure of the gut lining. Bone broth, which is rich in collagen and amino acids like glutamine, supports the repair of the intestinal lining, helping restore gut integrity.

Incorporating fermented foods like sauerkraut, kimchi, and kombucha introduces beneficial probiotics that promote a healthy gut microbiome. A diverse and balanced microbiome is essential for maintaining gut health, as it aids digestion, supports the immune system, and protects against harmful pathogens. A healthy gut microbiome also produces short-chain fatty acids (SCFAs) that help maintain the integrity of the gut lining and reduce inflammation. Improved gut integrity can enhance nutrient absorption, reduce gastrointestinal symptoms like bloating and gas, and decrease the immune system's exposure to potential triggers, thereby supporting overall digestive health.

Enhanced Energy Levels and Overall Well-being
Chronic inflammation and poor nutrient absorption can lead to fatigue and a general sense of unwellness in individuals with autoimmune conditions. The AIP diet emphasizes foods rich in essential vitamins, minerals, and antioxidants, providing the body with the nutrients it needs for optimal function. Many people experience increased energy levels and improved mental clarity by eliminating inflammatory foods and supporting gut health.

Stable blood sugar levels from consuming balanced, whole-food meals can prevent energy crashes and mood swings. Inflammatory foods, such as refined sugars and grains, can cause rapid spikes and drops in blood sugar, leading to energy fluctuations and irritability. The AIP diet promotes stable energy levels throughout the day by focusing on low-glycemic, nutrient-dense foods. This not only enhances physical energy but also improves mental clarity and focus.

The diet's focus on omega-3 fatty acids and antioxidants may also support brain health and reduce symptoms like brain fog. Brain fog is a common symptom of autoimmune conditions characterized by difficulty concentrating, memory issues, and mental fatigue. The anti-inflammatory properties of omega-3s, combined with the neuroprotective effects of antioxidants, can help reduce inflammation in the brain, leading to improved cognitive function. These dietary changes can contribute to better sleep quality, enhanced mood, and a greater overall sense of well-being, improving the quality of life for those following the AIP diet.

Supporting Weight Management and Hormonal Balance
The Paleo Autoimmune Protocol (AIP) Diet Cookbook offers many benefits for individuals seeking to manage autoimmune conditions and enhance overall health. The recipes are designed to promote gut healing by incorporating gut-soothing ingredients, which can

aid in repairing the gut lining and improving digestion. Eliminating inflammatory foods helps boost energy levels, reduce fatigue, and enhance vitality.

The AIP diet also supports weight management through balanced, anti-inflammatory meals that encourage healthy, gradual weight loss. The diet helps regulate metabolism and supports the body's natural detoxification processes by eliminating typical food triggers and focusing on whole, nutrient-dense foods. This can lead to a more balanced immune response and potentially reduce autoimmune flare-ups.

Focusing on whole, unprocessed foods and healthy fats also helps regulate hormones naturally, supporting hormonal balance. Many autoimmune conditions are linked to hormonal imbalances, particularly those involving the thyroid or adrenal glands. The AIP diet's emphasis on nutrient-rich foods helps support the endocrine system, promoting hormonal harmony and reducing symptoms associated with hormonal imbalances.

SUMMARY OF BENEFITS

Reduces Chronic Inflammation	The cookbook focuses on ingredients that help manage inflammation, which is crucial for autoimmune diseases.
Promotes Gut Healing	Recipes focus on gut-soothing ingredients, aiding in repairing the gut lining.
Boosts Energy Levels	It helps reduce fatigue and improve energy by eliminating inflammatory foods.
Improves Mental Clarity	Reduces brain fog and enhances cognitive function with brain-supporting nutrients.
Weight Management	Supports healthy, gradual weight loss through balanced, anti-inflammatory meals.
Balances Immune System	Aids in regulating the immune system by eliminating typical food triggers.
Customizable for Unique Needs	Flexible enough to combine with other diets, making it accessible for various dietary preferences.
Supports Hormonal Balance	Whole, unprocessed foods and healthy fats help naturally regulate hormones.
Enhances Skin Health	Promotes clearer, healthier skin by eliminating common skin-irritating triggers like dairy and refined sugars.
Sustainable Long-Term Success	Meal planning, reintroduction phases, and lifestyle tips provide long-term tools for sustaining the diet.
Holistic Approach to Healing	Includes stress and sleep management, offering a complete roadmap for physical and emotional health.

The Paleo Autoimmune Protocol (AIP) Diet Cookbook offers many benefits for individuals seeking to manage autoimmune conditions and enhance overall health. The cookbook addresses a fundamental aspect of autoimmune diseases by concentrating on ingredients that reduce chronic inflammation. The recipes are designed to promote gut healing by incorporating gut-soothing ingredients, which can aid in repairing the gut lining and improving digestion. Eliminating inflammatory foods helps boost energy levels, reduce fatigue, and enhance vitality. Including brain-supporting nutrients aims to improve mental clarity and reduce brain fog, contributing to better cognitive function.

The cookbook supports weight management through balanced, anti-inflammatory meals that encourage healthy, gradual weight loss. Eliminating typical food triggers aids in balancing the immune system, potentially reducing autoimmune flare-ups. Its flexibility allows customization to meet unique dietary needs, making it accessible for various preferences, including combinations with other diets like keto or vegetarian. Focusing on whole, unprocessed foods and healthy fats helps naturally regulate hormones, supporting hormonal balance. Additionally, eliminating common skin irritants such as dairy and refined sugars promotes clearer, healthier skin.

CHAPTER 2

The Science Behind AIP

The Autoimmune Protocol (AIP) diet is grounded in scientific principles addressing autoimmune diseases' root causes. By understanding the mechanisms of inflammation, gut health, and nutrient density, we can appreciate how the AIP diet supports healing and symptom management. This chapter delves into the science behind AIP, providing a foundation for its practical application.

2.1 Inflammation and Autoimmunity

Inflammation is the body's natural response to injury or infection, involving the immune system's deployment of white blood cells and chemical mediators to the affected area. While acute inflammation is protective, chronic inflammation can be detrimental, leading to tissue damage and contributing to various diseases, including autoimmune disorders.

In autoimmune diseases, the immune system mistakenly attacks the body's tissues, perpetuating a cycle of chronic inflammation. Factors contributing to this misdirected immune response include genetic predisposition, environmental triggers, and lifestyle factors such as diet.

Diet significantly influences inflammatory responses. Certain foods can exacerbate inflammation, such as:
- **Refined sugars and carbohydrates:** These can increase pro-inflammatory cytokines.
- **Trans fats and processed oils:** Found in many processed foods, they promote inflammation.
- **Food additives and preservatives:** They can trigger immune responses in sensitive individuals.

Conversely, anti-inflammatory foods can help modulate the immune system:
- **Omega-3 fatty acids:** Found in fatty fish like salmon, they reduce inflammation.
- **Antioxidant-rich fruits and vegetables:** They combat oxidative stress and inflammation.
- Spices like turmeric and ginger are known for their anti-inflammatory properties.

Studies support dietary intervention in managing autoimmune diseases. Research indicates that eliminating pro-inflammatory foods and incorporating anti-inflammatory nutrients can reduce disease activity and improve quality of life.

2.2 Gut Health Connection

The gut is essential for digestion and plays a pivotal role in immune function. The gut microbiome—a complex community of microorganisms—interacts with the immune system to maintain homeostasis. A healthy gut barrier prevents harmful substances from entering the bloodstream.

"Leaky gut" syndrome, or increased intestinal permeability, occurs when the gut lining becomes compromised. Factors contributing to leaky gut include:
- **Poor diet:** Consumption of gluten, alcohol, and processed foods can damage the gut lining.
- **Chronic stress:** It can alter gut microbiota and barrier function.
- **Medications:** NSAIDs (Nonsteroidal anti-inflammatory drugs) and antibiotics can disrupt gut integrity.

When the gut barrier is compromised, toxins, microbes, and undigested food particles can enter the bloodstream, triggering systemic inflammation and potentially initiating or exacerbating autoimmune responses.

The AIP diet focuses on healing the gut by:
- **Eliminating irritants:** Removing gluten, grains, legumes, dairy, and processed foods that may harm the gut lining.
- **Including gut-healing foods:** Bone broth provides collagen to repair the gut lining; fermented foods like sauerkraut introduce beneficial bacteria.
- **Supporting microbiome balance:** Prebiotic-rich vegetables like asparagus and garlic feed healthy gut bacteria.
- The AIP diet aims to reduce immune system overactivity and inflammation associated with autoimmune diseases by restoring gut integrity.

2.3 Nutrient Density and Healing

Autoimmune diseases often lead to nutrient deficiencies due to chronic inflammation, malabsorption, and increased nutrient demands. Essential nutrients support various bodily functions, including immune regulation, energy production, and tissue repair. Essential nutrients vital for healing include:

- **Vitamin D:** Modulates immune responses; deficiency is linked to increased autoimmune activity.
- **Zinc:** Essential for immune function and wound healing.
- **Selenium:** An antioxidant that protects cells from damage.

The AIP diet emphasizes nutrient-dense foods to replenish these critical nutrients:

- **Organ meats:** The liver and kidney are rich in vitamins A, B12, iron, and folate.
- **Seafood:** Provides omega-3 fatty acids, iodine, and selenium.
- **Colorful vegetables** Offer a wide range of vitamins, minerals, and antioxidants.

The AIP diet supports the body's natural healing processes by focusing on foods high in essential nutrients. Nutrient density accelerates recovery by:

- **Enhancing immune function:** Adequate nutrients help regulate the immune system.
- **Reducing oxidative stress:** Antioxidants neutralize free radicals that can damage cells.
- **Supporting tissue repair:** Proteins and minerals are crucial for rebuilding damaged tissues.

Understanding the science behind nutrient density reinforces the importance of food choices in managing autoimmune conditions.

By exploring the scientific foundations of inflammation, gut health, and nutrient density, we gain insight into how the AIP diet can positively impact autoimmune diseases. This knowledge empowers you to make informed decisions and fosters a more profound commitment to the dietary changes ahead. The next chapter will guide you through the practical steps of starting the AIP diet, ensuring a smooth transition toward better health.

2.4 The paleo autoimmune protocol (AIP) pyramid

The Paleo Autoimmune Protocol (AIP) Pyramid is a simplified visual guide designed to help individuals manage autoimmune conditions through diet. It adapts to the traditional Paleo diet, focusing on nutrient-dense foods while eliminating potential triggers that may cause inflammation. At the base of the pyramid, you'll find vegetables—primarily leafy greens, cruciferous vegetables, and root vegetables—forming the foundation of this anti-inflammatory diet. Above that, moderate portions of high-quality proteins like grass-fed meats, wild-caught fish, and organ meats are emphasized to support healing and immune function. Healthy fats, such as coconut oil, avocado, and olive oil, occupy the next level, providing essential nutrients for cell health and reducing inflammation. Small amounts of fermented foods, like sauerkraut or kombucha, are included for gut health, while fruits, such as berries, are recommended in moderation for antioxidants. The top of the pyramid represents herbs and spices used sparingly for their anti-inflammatory properties. Foods that are commonly inflammatory, like grains, dairy, legumes, nightshades, and processed foods, are eliminated in the Paleo AIP diet to promote overall healing and balance in the body.

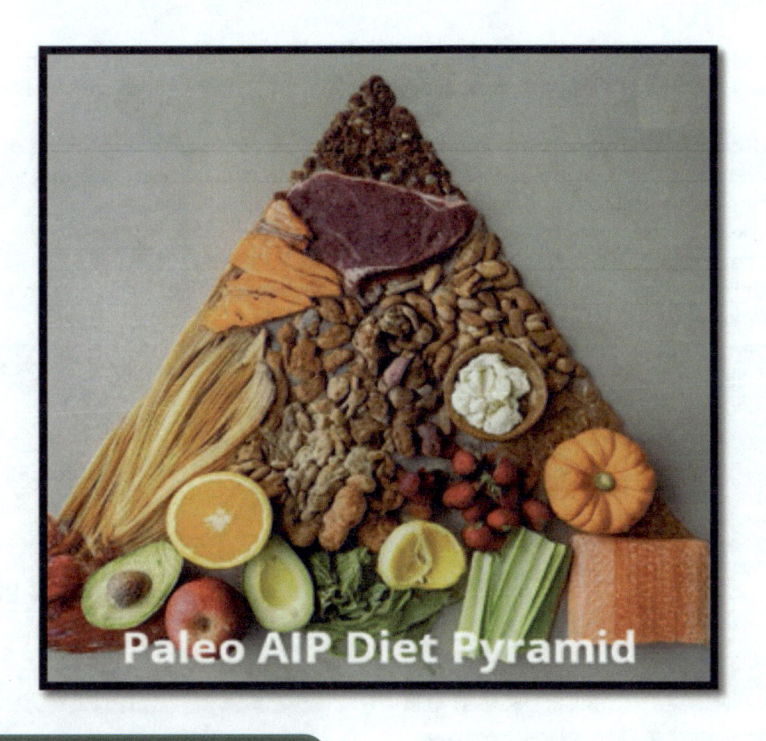

CHAPTER 3

Getting Started with AIP

Embarking on the Autoimmune Protocol (AIP) diet is a significant step toward managing autoimmune conditions and improving overall health. This chapter provides practical guidance on beginning your AIP journey, including which foods to eliminate, which to embrace, and strategies to ease the transition. By understanding these essential elements, you'll be well-equipped to implement the AIP diet effectively.

3.1 Foods to Eliminate

The elimination phase is the cornerstone of the AIP diet, aiming to reduce inflammation by removing foods that may trigger immune responses or irritate the gut. Here's a comprehensive list of foods to avoid:

- Grains: Wheat, barley, rye, oats, corn, rice, and all grain-derived products. Grains contain gluten and lectins, which can contribute to gut permeability and inflammation.
- Legumes: Beans, lentils, peas, peanuts, soy, and soy products. Legumes have proteins and antinutrients that may irritate the digestive system.
- Dairy: Milk, cheese, yogurt, butter, and all dairy derivatives. Dairy proteins like casein can provoke immune reactions in sensitive individuals.
- Nightshade Vegetables: Tomatoes, potatoes (excluding sweet potatoes), eggplants, peppers, and spices like paprika and cayenne. Nightshades contain alkaloids that may exacerbate inflammation.
- Nuts and Seeds: All nuts and seeds, including foods made from them like nut butter and seed oils. They can be challenging to digest and may cause immune reactions.
- Eggs: Both egg whites and yolks are eliminated due to potential allergenic proteins.
- Processed Foods: Foods with additives, preservatives, refined sugars, and artificial sweeteners. These can trigger inflammation and disrupt gut health.
- Alcohol and Caffeine: Both can irritate the gut lining and affect the immune system.

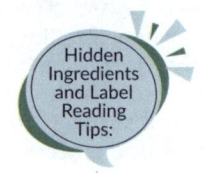

Hidden Ingredients and Label Reading Tips: Many processed foods contain hidden sources of eliminated items. For example, soy and dairy derivatives may appear in sauces and dressings, while gluten can be in spice mixes. Reading labels carefully is essential. Look for keywords like maltodextrin (often derived from corn), casein (a milk protein), and natural flavors (which can include a variety of non-AIP ingredients). When in doubt, opt for whole, unprocessed foods to ensure compliance.

3.2 Foods to Enjoy

The AIP diet emphasizes nutrient-dense, anti-inflammatory foods that support healing. Here's what you can enjoy:

- Meats and Poultry: Grass-fed beef, lamb, pork, free-range chicken, and turkey. Organ meats like liver and heart are particularly nutrient-rich.
- Fish and Seafood: Wild-caught fish (salmon, mackerel) and shellfish (shrimp, oysters) provide omega-3 fatty acids.
- Vegetables: A wide variety, excluding nightshades. Leafy greens (spinach, kale), cruciferous vegetables (broccoli, cauliflower), root vegetables (carrots, sweet potatoes), and squashes.
- Fruits: In moderation, focusing on lower-sugar options like berries, apples, and pears.
- Healthy Fats: Olive oil, coconut oil, avocado oil, and animal fats like lard and tallow.
- Herbs and Spices: Fresh herbs (basil, rosemary, thyme) and non-seed spices like garlic, ginger, and turmeric.
- Fermented Foods: Sauerkraut, kombucha, and coconut yogurt for probiotics.

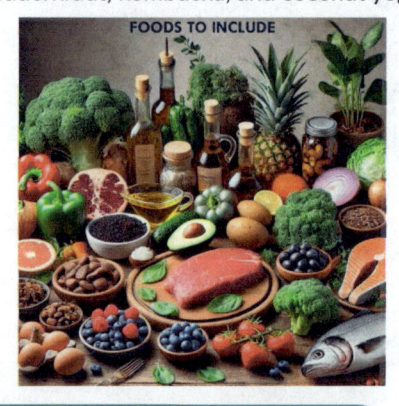

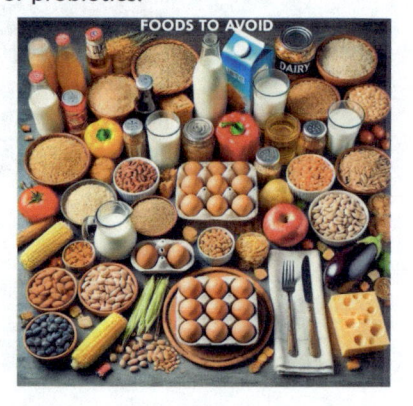

Emphasis on Variety and Nutrient-Rich Choices:
Incorporating a diverse range of foods ensures you receive essential vitamins and minerals. For example, leafy greens are rich in magnesium and calcium, while seafood provides iodine and selenium. Variety also keeps meals exciting and satisfying, reducing the temptation to revert to non-compliant foods.

Seasonal Eating and Sourcing Quality Ingredients:
Eating seasonally available produce enhances nutrient intake and freshness. Visiting local farmers' markets can provide access to organic and sustainably raised foods. Prioritize high-quality sources, such as grass-fed meats and organic vegetables, to minimize exposure to pesticides and hormones

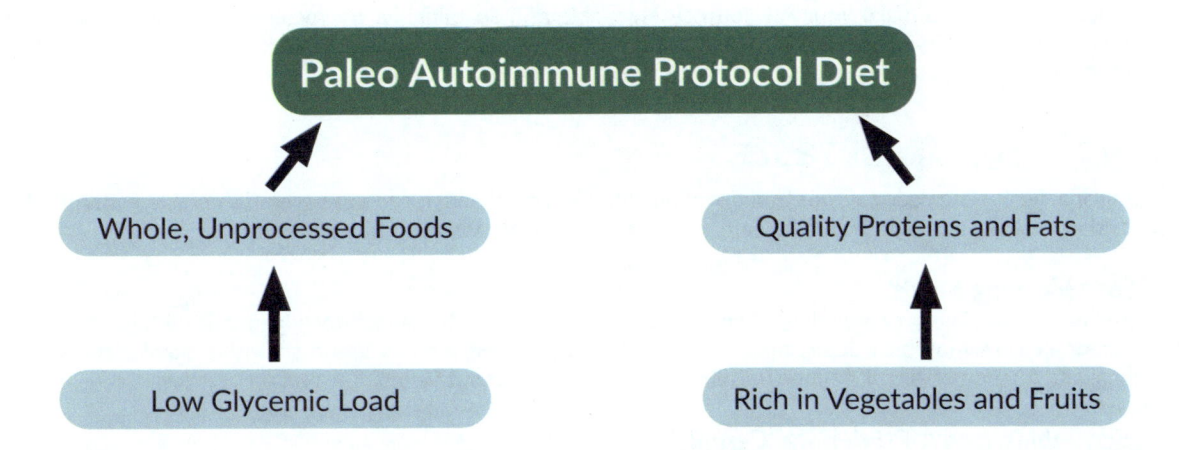

```
                    Paleo Autoimmune Protocol Diet
                              ↑         ↑
            Whole, Unprocessed Foods   Quality Proteins and Fats
                       ↑                        ↑
              Low Glycemic Load        Rich in Vegetables and Fruits
```

3.3 Transition Strategies

Adopting the AIP diet can be a significant lifestyle change. Here are strategies to facilitate a smooth transition:

- **Planning and Preparing Your Kitchen:**
  - **Pantry Audit:** Remove non-compliant foods to reduce temptation.
  - **Stock Up on Essentials:** Fill your pantry and fridge with AIP-friendly staples like fresh vegetables, meats, and approved cooking oils.
  - **Meal Planning:** Create a weekly meal plan to streamline shopping and cooking.

- **Tips for Easing into the Diet:**
  - **Gradual Elimination:** If diving in all at once feels overwhelming, consider eliminating one food category at a time.
  - **Simple Recipes:** Start with straightforward recipes that require minimal ingredients and steps.
  - **Focus on Additions:** Instead of fixating on what you're eliminating, focus on the new, delicious foods you're incorporating.

- **Overcoming Common Challenges and Cravings:**
  - **Cravings:** Combat cravings by ensuring satisfying meals incorporate healthy fats and proteins to promote satiety.
  - **Social Situations:** Plan for dining out or attending events by researching restaurants or bringing AIP-compliant dishes to share.
  - **Mindset and Support:** Maintain a positive outlook and seek support from friends, family, or online AIP communities.

Managing Expectations:
It's essential to recognize that adjustments may take time. You might experience withdrawal symptoms or emotional responses as your body adapts. Patience and self-compassion are key. Remember that the elimination phase is temporary; the ultimate goal is identifying the foods that work best for your body.

By understanding which foods to eliminate and embrace and implementing effective transition strategies, you're setting a solid foundation for success on the AIP diet. This proactive approach empowers you to take control of your health, reduce inflammation, and potentially alleviate symptoms associated with autoimmune conditions. The next chapter will provide a collection of delicious AIP recipes to support and enhance your culinary journey.

CHAPTER 4

Delicious AIP Recipes

Embarking on the Autoimmune Protocol (AIP) diet doesn't mean sacrificing flavor or variety. This chapter introduces a collection of delicious recipes designed to make your AIP journey enjoyable and sustainable. By focusing on wholesome, nutrient-dense ingredients, you can create satisfying meals that comply with AIP guidelines. From energizing breakfasts to hearty lunches, dinners, and satisfying snacks and treats, these recipes nourish your body and delight your palate.

4.1 Energizing Breakfasts

Breakfast is essential for fueling your day, but traditional options like cereal, toast, and eggs are off the table with AIP. However, this opens up a world of creative and nutritious alternatives that can invigorate your mornings.

Quick and Easy Morning Meals
For those rushed mornings, simplicity is vital. A warm bowl of apple-cinnamon breakfast porridge made with grated apples, coconut milk, and a sprinkle of cinnamon provides comfort and energy. Another option is a green smoothie bowl blended with spinach, avocado, banana, and a touch of ginger, topped with fresh berries and coconut flakes.

Smoothies, Scrambles, and AIP-Friendly "Cereals"
- **Smoothies:** These are a fantastic way to pack in nutrients quickly. Try blending mango, pineapple, and leafy greens with coconut water for a tropical boost. Adding collagen peptides can enhance protein content and support gut health.
- **Scrambles:** While eggs are eliminated, you can create a satisfying breakfast scramble using ground turkey or beef sautéed with onions, bell pepper substitutes like diced zucchini, and fresh herbs like basil and oregano.
- **AIP-Friendly "Cereals":** Create a grain-free cereal by mixing shredded coconut, sliced bananas, and chopped tiger nuts (a tuber resembling nuts) drizzled with coconut milk. This combination offers texture and natural sweetness.

Batch Cooking for Busy Mornings
Preparing breakfasts ahead of time can alleviate morning stress. Consider making:
- **Breakfast Patties:** Mix ground meat with grated vegetables like carrots and zucchini, season with AIP-friendly spices, form into patties, and cook in batches. Freeze portions for quick reheating.
- **Baked Sweet Potato Toasts:** Slice sweet potatoes lengthwise, bake until tender, and store in the fridge. In the morning, top with avocado mash and smoked salmon for a nutritious meal.
- **Overnight Chia Pudding:** Soak chia seeds in coconut milk overnight with a dash of vanilla extract. In the morning, top with fresh fruit for a fiber-rich breakfast.

4.2 Hearty Lunches and Dinners

Lunches and dinners are opportunities to enjoy robust flavors and various textures. By combining proteins with an array of vegetables and herbs, you can create meals that are both healing and hearty.

Satisfying Soups, Stews, and Main Dishes
- **Soups and Stews:** These dishes are easily adaptable and ideal for batch cooking. A comforting bowl of butternut squash soup blended with coconut milk and seasoned with nutmeg warms the soul. Alternatively, a seafood stew with shrimp, cod, and mussels simmered in a broth with garlic, fennel, and saffron offers a taste of the Mediterranean.
- **Main Dishes:** Enjoy grilled grass-fed steak topped with a chimichurri sauce made from parsley, garlic, and olive oil, accompanied by roasted Brussels sprouts. Baked chicken thighs marinated in lemon juice, rosemary, and olive oil served with cauliflower "rice" make for a satisfying meal.

Incorporating Variety with Proteins and Vegetables
Diversity in your diet not only prevents boredom but also ensures a broad spectrum of nutrients:
- **Proteins:** Rotate between different meats like bison, duck, and rabbit. Incorporate seafood such as scallops and clams for variety and additional minerals like zinc and iodine.
- **Vegetables:** Explore less common vegetables like kohlrabi, artichokes, and collard greens. Each offers unique flavors and nutritional benefits.
- **Flavor Enhancers:** Use fresh herbs, citrus juices, and AIP-compliant spices to elevate dishes. A squeeze of lemon or a sprinkle of fresh dill can transform a meal.

One-Pot Meals and Slow Cooker Recipes
One-pot and slow cooker recipes save time and infuse dishes with deep flavors:
- **One-Pot Meals:** A hearty ratatouille using AIP-approved vegetables like zucchini, squash, and carrots simmered in a tomato-free sauce makes for a nourishing meal. Add ground meat for extra protein.
- **Slow Cooker Recipes:** Prepare a tender beef brisket with root vegetables like parsnips and turnips. Let it cook slowly with broth, garlic, and bay leaves for a melt-in-your-mouth experience.
- **Sheet Pan Dinners:** Arrange chicken pieces and a medley of vegetables on a sheet pan, drizzle with olive oil and herbs, and roast for an easy cleanup meal.

4.3 Snacks and Treats

Snacking doesn't have to be mundane on the AIP diet. You can enjoy satisfying snacks and treats that align with your dietary needs with a bit of creativity.

Portable Snacks for On-the-Go
- **Dehydrated Snacks:** Make your vegetable chips using kale, zucchini, or beetroot. Season with sea salt and bake or dehydrate until crisp.
- **Meat Sticks and Jerky:** Prepare homemade meat sticks using ground meat seasoned with compliant spices, which are formed into sticks and dehydrated. They offer a convenient protein boost.
- **Fruit Leather:** Puree fruits like apples and strawberries, spread thinly on parchment paper, and dehydrate to create natural fruit rolls.

Healthy Alternatives to Favorite Treats
- **Gelatin Gummies:** Use grass-fed gelatin, fruit purees, and a touch of honey to make chewy gummies rich in gut-healing gelatin.
- **Baked Goods:** Create AIP-friendly muffins using green plantains or cassava flour as a base, sweetened with mashed bananas or applesauce.
- **Mock Chocolate Treats:** Carob powder can substitute cocoa in recipes, allowing you to enjoy "chocolate" pudding or carob chip cookies without caffeine.

Mindful Indulgences Without Compromising the Diet
Enjoying treats mindfully ensures you don't feel deprived:
- **Portion Control:** Serve treats in small portions to savor the flavors without overindulging.
- **Mindful Eating Practices:** Eat without distractions, focusing on the taste, texture, and aroma of your food. This enhances satisfaction and can prevent overeating.
- **Occasional Indulgence:** Allow yourself an occasional AIP-compliant treat to maintain balance. This can help sustain long-term adherence to the diet.

Hydration and Beverages
Don't overlook the importance of beverages:
- **Herbal Teas:** Enjoy teas made from chamomile, peppermint, or rooibos. They can be soothing and offer health benefits.
- **Infused Waters:** Add slices of cucumber, berries, or citrus fruits to water for a refreshing drink.
- **Broths:** Sipping bone broth between meals can provide additional nutrients and support gut health.

You can make the AIP diet enjoyable and nourishing by embracing these recipes and meal ideas. Cooking at home gives you complete control over ingredients, ensuring compliance with the diet while catering to your tastes. Remember, variety and creativity are your allies in maintaining enthusiasm and satisfaction with your meals. The following chapter will delve into sustaining and personalizing your AIP journey for long-term success.

VEGETABLES

Leafy Greens	Kale, Spinach, Swiss Chard, Collard Greens, Arugula, Romaine Lettuce
Cruciferous Vegetables	Broccoli, Cauliflower, Brussels Sprouts, Cabbage, Bok Choy
Root Vegetables	Sweet Potatoes, Carrots, Beets, Parsnips, Rutabaga, Turnips
Squash Varieties	Zucchini, Butternut Squash, Spaghetti Squash, Acorn Squash
Other Vegetables	Cucumber, Asparagus, Celery, Leeks, Fennel, Green Beans (in moderation), Artichokes
Herbs	Parsley, Cilantro, Basil, Thyme, Oregano, Rosemary

These vegetables are anti-inflammatory, nutrient-dense, and free from common food triggers that the AIP diet avoids. It's essential to avoid nightshades, such as tomatoes, potatoes, eggplants, and peppers, as they can trigger autoimmune symptoms.

HEALING FOODS

Bone Broths	Chicken Bone Broth, Beef Bone Broth, Fish Bone Broth, Lamb Bone Broth, Turkey Bone Broth
Pastured Meats and Wild-Caught Fish	Grass-fed beef, Pastured Chicken, Pastured Pork, Grass-Fed Lamb, Pastured Turkey, Wild-Caught Salmon, Wild-Caught Mackerel, Wild-Caught Sardines, Wild-Caught Cod, Venison (Deer), Bison
Healthy Fats	Coconut Oil, Olive Oil (Extra Virgin), Avocado Oil, Lard (from pasture-raised animals), Tallow (from grass-fed animals), Duck Fat, Coconut Milk (unsweetened), Palm Oil (sustainably sourced), Ghee (if tolerated)
Fruit (in moderation)	Berries (Blueberries, Raspberries, Strawberries, Blackberries), Apples, Pears, Mangoes, Peaches, Plums, Bananas (especially green bananas), Pineapple, Watermelon, Papaya
Herbs and Spices	Basil, Parsley, Thyme, Rosemary, Oregano, Sage, Turmeric (anti-inflammatory), Ginger (anti-inflammatory), Garlic, Cinnamon, Cloves, Tarragon, Cilantro, Dill, Marjoram, Lemongrass, Bay Leaves
Baking Ingredients	Coconut Flour, Cassava Flour, Arrowroot Flour, Tigernut Flour, Sweet Potato Flour, Green Banana Flour, Tapioca Starch
Sweeteners (in moderation)	Raw Honey, Maple Syrup, Molasses, Date Syrup
Other Healing Foods	Fermented Foods (Sauerkraut, Kimchi made without nightshades, Coconut Yogurt), Sea Vegetables (Nori, Kelp, Dulse, Wakame), Gelatin and Collagen Peptides (Grass-Fed), Coconut Aminos (soy sauce alternative), Nutritional Yeast (if tolerated), Organ Meats (Liver, Heart, Kidney, from grass-fed animals), Shellfish (Shrimp, Lobster, Crab, Mussels, Oysters)

These foods are nutrient-dense, support gut health, and help reduce inflammation, which is critical for those following the AIP diet for autoimmune healing.

CHAPTER 5

Sustaining and Personalizing Your AIP Journey

Embarking on the Autoimmune Protocol (AIP) diet is a significant step toward managing autoimmune conditions, but the journey doesn't end with the elimination phase. Sustaining the diet and personalizing it to suit your needs is crucial for long-term success and overall well-being. This chapter explores how to navigate the reintroduction phase, the importance of lifestyle factors, and strategies for maintaining progress over time.

5.1 The Reintroduction Phase

The reintroduction phase is a systematic process of gradually adding eliminated foods back into your diet to identify specific triggers. This phase is essential for personalizing the AIP diet to your unique tolerances and ensuring nutritional adequacy.

When and How to Reintroduce Foods
After adhering strictly to the elimination phase for at least 30 to 90 days—or until you notice a significant improvement in symptoms—you can reintroduce foods. The process involves:
1. **Choosing a Single Food:** Select one food to reintroduce, starting with items less likely to cause reactions, such as egg yolks or certain nuts.
2. **Gradual Testing:** Consume a small amount (e.g., a teaspoon) and monitor for immediate reactions. If none occur, increase the portion to a tablespoon later in the day and then to a standard serving the next day.
3. **Observation Period:** Wait 3 to 7 days before introducing another food, as some reactions can be delayed.

Tracking Reactions and Symptoms
Keeping a detailed food diary is crucial during this phase. Record:
- **Foods Reintroduced:** Note the type, amount, and time of consumption.
- **Symptoms Experienced:** Monitor for digestive issues, joint pain, skin reactions, fatigue, or mood changes.
- **Overall Well-being:** Assess energy levels, sleep quality, and emotional state.

This meticulous tracking helps identify which foods are well-tolerated and which may need to remain excluded.

Adjusting the Diet Based on Individual Responses
The reintroduction phase allows you to tailor the AIP diet to your body's responses. If a food doesn't cause adverse reactions, it can be reintegrated into your regular diet, broadening your nutritional options. Conversely, if symptoms reappear, it's advisable to eliminate that food and possibly retest it later.

5.2 Lifestyle Factors

Diet is fundamental to managing autoimmune conditions, but addressing lifestyle factors influencing immune function and inflammation is equally essential.

Stress Management Techniques
Chronic stress can exacerbate autoimmune symptoms by triggering inflammatory pathways. Effective stress management strategies include:
- **Mindfulness and Meditation:** Practicing mindfulness helps reduce stress and improve emotional resilience.
- **Deep Breathing Exercises:** Techniques like diaphragmatic breathing can calm the nervous system.
- **Time Management:** Prioritizing tasks and setting realistic goals prevent being overwhelmed.

Importance of Sleep and Relaxation
Adequate sleep is vital for immune regulation and tissue repair. Aim for 7-9 hours of quality sleep per night by:
- **Establishing a Sleep Routine:** Go to bed and wake up at consistent times.
- **Creating a Restful Environment:** Ensure your bedroom is dark, quiet, and cool.
- **Limiting Screen Time:** Avoid electronic devices at least an hour before bedtime.

Incorporating Exercise and Physical Activity
Regular physical activity supports overall health but should be balanced to avoid overexertion, which can trigger flare-ups.
- **Gentle Exercises:** Walking, yoga, and swimming are low-impact and can improve circulation and flexibility.

- **Listening to Your Body:** Adjust intensity based on feelings, allowing rest when needed.
- **Consistency Over Intensity:** Regular moderate exercise is more beneficial than sporadic intense workouts.

5.3 Long-Term Success and Support

Sustaining the AIP diet and lifestyle changes requires ongoing commitment and support.
Building a Supportive Community
Connecting with others who understand your journey can provide encouragement and accountability.
- **Join Support Groups:** Online forums and local meetups offer platforms to share experiences and tips.
- **Involve Family and Friends:** Educate loved ones about your dietary needs to gain their support.
- **Work with Professionals:** Dietitians, nutritionists, and health coaches specialized in AIP can offer personalized guidance.

Resources for Continued Learning
Staying informed empowers you to make better choices.
- **Educational Materials:** Books, reputable websites, and scientific articles deepen your understanding of autoimmune health.
- **Cooking Classes and Workshops:** Learn new recipes and cooking techniques to keep meals exciting.
- **Podcasts and Webinars:** Accessible formats to stay updated on the latest research and strategies.

Adapting the AIP Diet for Lifelong Health
The AIP diet may evolve to suit your changing needs as you progress.
- **Periodic Re-evaluation:** Regularly assess your symptoms and dietary tolerances to adjust accordingly.
- **Maintenance Phase:** Establish a balanced diet that includes a variety of foods you tolerate well.
- **Holistic Approach:** Integrate diet with lifestyle practices for comprehensive health management.

By embracing the reintroduction phase, addressing key lifestyle factors, and seeking support, you can effectively sustain and personalize the AIP diet. This holistic approach not only aids in managing autoimmune symptoms but also promotes long-term health and vitality. Remember, the journey is personal, and patience with yourself is paramount. Celebrate your progress, learn from setbacks, and nurture your body and mind for optimal well-being.

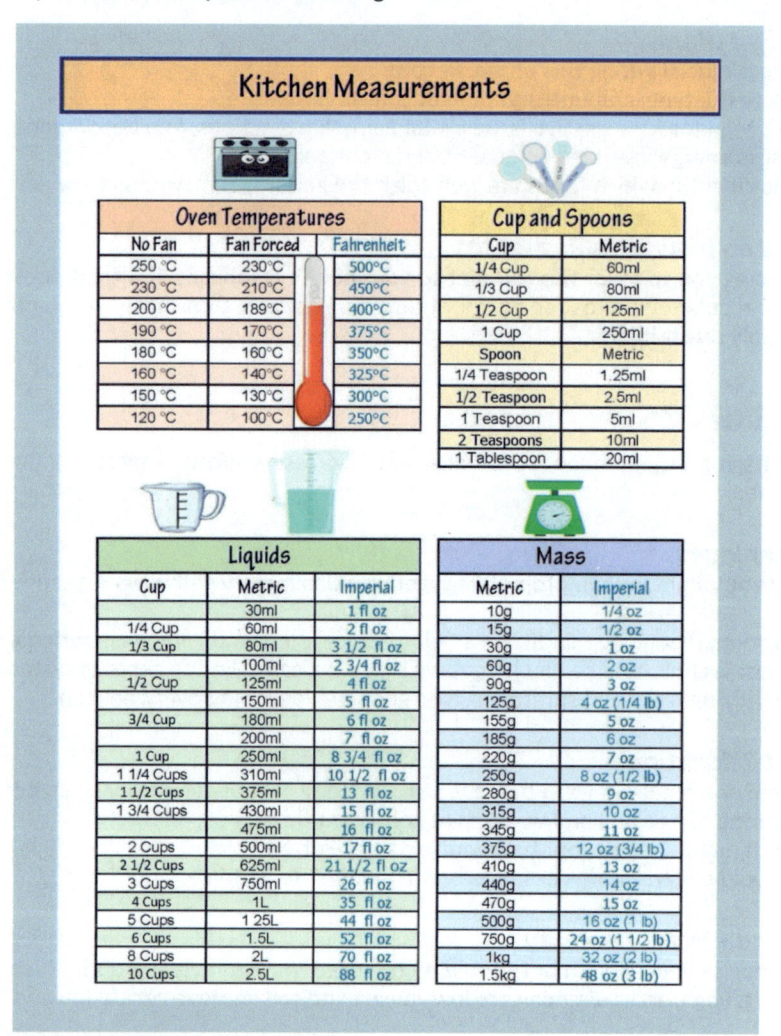

Kitchen Measurements

Oven Temperatures

No Fan	Fan Forced	Fahrenheit
250 °C	230°C	500°C
230 °C	210°C	450°C
200 °C	189°C	400°C
190 °C	170°C	375°C
180 °C	160°C	350°C
160 °C	140°C	325°C
150 °C	130°C	300°C
120 °C	100°C	250°C

Cup and Spoons

Cup	Metric
1/4 Cup	60ml
1/3 Cup	80ml
1/2 Cup	125ml
1 Cup	250ml
Spoon	Metric
1/4 Teaspoon	1.25ml
1/2 Teaspoon	2.5ml
1 Teaspoon	5ml
2 Teaspoons	10ml
1 Tablespoon	20ml

Liquids

Cup	Metric	Imperial
	30ml	1 fl oz
1/4 Cup	60ml	2 fl oz
1/3 Cup	80ml	3 1/2 fl oz
	100ml	2 3/4 fl oz
1/2 Cup	125ml	4 fl oz
	150ml	5 fl oz
3/4 Cup	180ml	6 fl oz
	200ml	7 fl oz
1 Cup	250ml	8 3/4 fl oz
1 1/4 Cups	310ml	10 1/2 fl oz
1 1/2 Cups	375ml	13 fl oz
1 3/4 Cups	430ml	15 fl oz
	475ml	16 fl oz
2 Cups	500ml	17 fl oz
2 1/2 Cups	625ml	21 1/2 fl oz
3 Cups	750ml	26 fl oz
4 Cups	1L	35 fl oz
5 Cups	1.25L	44 fl oz
6 Cups	1.5L	52 fl oz
8 Cups	2L	70 fl oz
10 Cups	2.5L	88 fl oz

Mass

Metric	Imperial
10g	1/4 oz
15g	1/2 oz
30g	1 oz
60g	2 oz
90g	3 oz
125g	4 oz (1/4 lb)
155g	5 oz
185g	6 oz
220g	7 oz
250g	8 oz (1/2 lb)
280g	9 oz
315g	10 oz
345g	11 oz
375g	12 oz (3/4 lb)
410g	13 oz
440g	14 oz
470g	15 oz
500g	16 oz (1 lb)
750g	24 oz (1 1/2 lb)
1kg	32 oz (2 lb)
1.5kg	48 oz (3 lb)

Frequently Asked Questions (F.A.Q.)

Here are some of the most common questions regarding the Paleo Autoimmune Protocol (AIP) Diet and the cookbook, along with detailed answers to help guide you on your journey to better health.

1. What is the Paleo Autoimmune Protocol (AIP) Diet, and how does it differ from the standard Paleo diet?
The Paleo Autoimmune Protocol (AIP) diet is a more restrictive version of the standard Paleo diet, specifically designed to help manage autoimmune diseases by reducing inflammation, promoting gut healing, and balancing the immune system. While the standard Paleo diet eliminates grains, legumes, dairy, processed foods, and refined sugars, the AIP diet also removes nuts, seeds, nightshade vegetables (like tomatoes, peppers, and eggplants), eggs, and certain spices. The AIP diet focuses on nutrient-dense foods such as grass-fed meats, wild-caught fish, non-nightshade vegetables, healthy fats, bone broth, and fermented foods to support gut health and reduce inflammation.

2. Who can benefit from following the AIP diet?
The AIP diet is particularly beneficial for individuals with autoimmune conditions such as rheumatoid arthritis, lupus, Hashimoto's thyroiditis, Crohn's disease, celiac disease, and multiple sclerosis, among others. It can also help those with chronic inflammation, digestive disorders, and food sensitivities. The AIP diet aims to reduce symptoms, improve gut health, and promote well-being by eliminating potential food triggers and focusing on nutrient-dense, anti-inflammatory foods. However, it's essential to consult with a healthcare professional before starting the AIP diet, especially if you have underlying health conditions.

3. How long should I follow the AIP diet, and when can I start reintroducing foods?
The AIP diet is typically followed in two phases: the elimination phase and the reintroduction phase. The elimination phase, where you avoid all potentially inflammatory foods, usually lasts 30-60 days. During this period, you focus on healing the gut and reducing inflammation. After the elimination phase, you can start the reintroduction phase, where you slowly reintroduce eliminated foods one at a time while monitoring your body's response to identify any food sensitivities or triggers. This process lets you personalize your diet and determine which foods you can tolerate. Being patient and systematic during the reintroduction phase is essential to avoid potential flare-ups.

4. What foods are allowed and not allowed on the AIP diet?
Allowed foods on the AIP diet include grass-fed meats, wild-caught fish, pasture-raised poultry, organ meats, non-nightshade vegetables (like leafy greens, cruciferous vegetables, and root vegetables), healthy fats (such as olive oil, coconut oil, and avocado oil), bone broth, fermented foods (like sauerkraut and kimchi without nightshades), coconut-based products, and AIP-compliant herbs and spices. Foods that are not allowed include grains, legumes, dairy, refined sugars, nuts, seeds, nightshade vegetables (such as tomatoes, peppers, and eggplants), eggs, processed foods, and certain spices like paprika and cumin.

5. How does the AIP diet help in managing autoimmune diseases?
The AIP diet helps manage autoimmune diseases by reducing inflammation, promoting gut health, and supporting immune system balance. Autoimmune conditions often involve a leaky gut, where the gut lining becomes permeable, allowing undigested food particles and toxins to enter the bloodstream, triggering an immune response. The AIP diet eliminates common inflammatory foods and focuses on gut-healing foods like bone broth, fermented vegetables, and fiber-rich produce, which help repair the gut lining, reduce inflammation, and prevent flare-ups.

6. Are there any side effects when starting the AIP diet?
When starting the AIP diet, some people may experience initial side effects, such as fatigue, headaches, irritability, and cravings, commonly known as "detox" or "withdrawal" symptoms. These occur as your body adjusts to removing inflammatory foods, refined sugars, and processed ingredients. These symptoms are typically temporary and may last a few days to a week. To minimize discomfort, stay hydrated, get plenty of rest, and focus on nutrient-dense foods to support your body during this transition.

7. What should I expect from the AIP cookbook regarding meal variety and recipes?
The AIP cookbook offers various delicious, nutrient-dense recipes that cater to different tastes and preferences while adhering to AIP guidelines. It includes breakfast options like smoothies and breakfast bowls, lunch ideas such as hearty salads and protein-packed wraps, dinner recipes including one-pot meals and international cuisines, snacks, sides, desserts, and beverages. Each recipe uses AIP-compliant ingredients to ensure a well-rounded, flavorful, and healing meal experience.

8. Can I follow the AIP diet if I have other dietary restrictions or preferences (e.g., vegetarian, low-FODMAP, keto)?
The AIP diet can be adapted to accommodate other dietary restrictions or preferences. However, it may require more planning and creativity to ensure you are getting adequate nutrition. For example, if you follow a vegetarian or low-FODMAP diet, focus on non-nightshade vegetables, fruits, coconut-based products, and AIP-friendly plant-based proteins like fermented vegetables and certain seeds (if tolerated). You can combine AIP principles with high-fat, low-carb ingredients like avocados, coconut oil, and fatty fish for those on a keto diet. Always consult a healthcare professional or dietitian to ensure you meet your nutritional needs.

9. How do I stay motivated and manage cravings while on the AIP diet?

Staying motivated on the AIP diet can be challenging, especially when cravings arise. Eat balanced meals with adequate protein, healthy fats, and fiber to manage cravings. Keep AIP-friendly snacks, such as plantain chips, coconut-date energy bites, and bone broth. Meal planning, preparation, and finding creative ways to enjoy favorite flavors within the AIP framework can also help. Remember that cravings often diminish as your body adjusts to the diet, and focusing on your health goals can help keep you motivated.

10. Is the AIP diet suitable for long-term use?

The AIP diet is not intended to be a long-term, permanent diet. Instead, it is a short-term intervention to help identify food sensitivities and promote healing. Once you have completed the elimination and reintroduction phases and identified your personal food triggers, you can transition to a maintenance phase that includes a broader range of well-tolerated foods. However, some individuals may maintain aspects of the AIP diet long-term to support ongoing health and wellness, especially if they experience benefits.

These FAQs provide a comprehensive understanding of the Paleo Autoimmune Protocol Diet and what to expect from following the guidelines outlined in the cookbook. By addressing common concerns and providing practical advice, anyone interested in the AIP diet can feel more confident and prepared to embark on this healing journey.

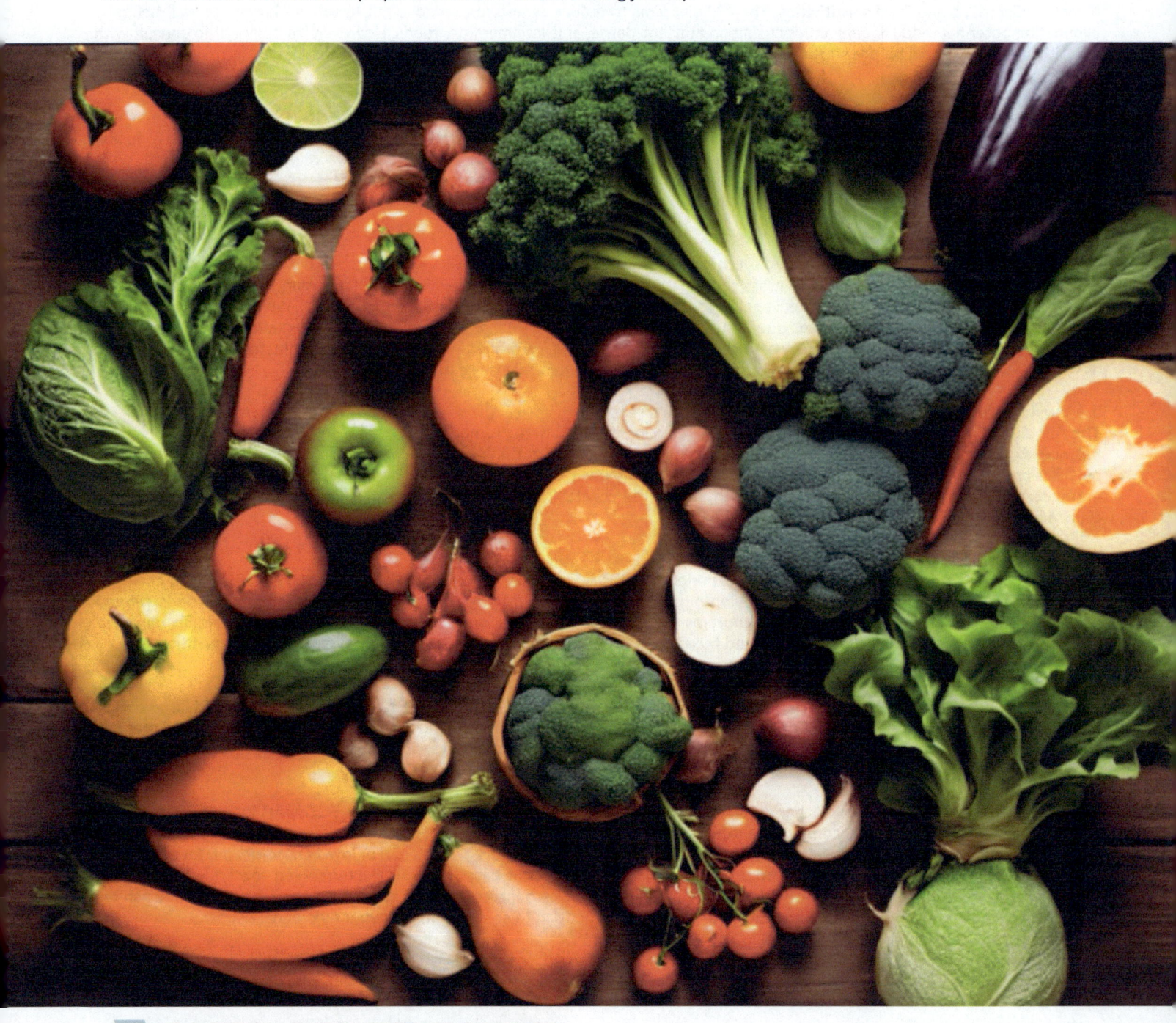

CHAPTER 6: AIP BREAKFAST RECIPES

1. Green Gut-Healing Smoothie

Yield: 1 serving | Prep Time: 5 minutes | Cooking Time: None | Total Time: 5 minutes | Difficulty Level: Easy

Description: This refreshing, nutrient-packed smoothie combines greens, healthy fats, and hydrating coconut water to support gut health. It is perfect for a light breakfast or snack to aid digestion.

Ingredients:
- 30g fresh spinach (1 cup)
- 60g cucumber, chopped (½ cup)
- 80g pineapple chunks, fresh or frozen (½ cup)
- ½ avocado
- 15g grated fresh ginger (1 tablespoon)
- 15ml coconut oil (1 tablespoon)
- 240ml coconut water (1 cup)
- 15g collagen peptides (optional, 1 tablespoon)
- Juice of ½ lemon
- 1 cup fresh spinach
- ½ cup cucumber, chopped
- ½ cup pineapple chunks (fresh or frozen)
- ½ avocado
- 1 tablespoon grated fresh ginger
- 1 tablespoon coconut oil
- 1 cup coconut water
- 1 tablespoon collagen peptides (optional)
- Juice of ½ lemon

Instructions:
1. Add all ingredients to a blender.
2. Blend on high until smooth and creamy.
3. Pour into a glass and enjoy immediately.

Dietary Main Goals:
Gut Health Support – Weight Loss

Storage & Reheating:
Best served fresh. If storing, refrigerate in a sealed container for up to 24 hours. Stir or shake well before drinking if stored.

Budget-Friendly Notes:
Using frozen pineapple can reduce costs without sacrificing flavor or nutrition.
Serving Size: 1 smoothie (about 350ml)

Nutrition Information: (Per Serving)
- Calories: 220 kcal
- Protein: 5g
- Carbohydrates: 18g
- Fiber: 7g
- Sugars: 9g
- Fat: 16g

2. Berry Coconut Breakfast Bowl

Yield: 1 serving | Prep Time: 5 minutes | Cooking Time: None | Total Time: 5 minutes | Difficulty Level: Easy

Description: A delicious and creamy breakfast bowl of mixed berries and AIP-compliant coconut yogurt, topped with chia seeds and coconut flakes. This bowl is a perfect way to start the day with a nutritious boost.

Ingredients:
- 150g / 1 cup mixed berries (blueberries, raspberries, blackberries)
- 120g / ½ cup coconut yogurt (AIP-compliant)
- 7g / 1 tablespoon shredded coconut
- 10g / 1 tablespoon chia seeds
- 7g / 1 tablespoon unsweetened coconut flakes
- 15g / 1 tablespoon pumpkin seed butter (optional)
- 5ml / 1 teaspoon honey or maple syrup (optional)

Instructions:
1. In a bowl, mix coconut yogurt and chia seeds. Let it sit for 5 minutes to thicken.
2. Top with mixed berries, shredded coconut, and coconut flakes.
3. Drizzle with honey or maple syrup if desired.
4. Serve immediately.

Dietary Main Goals:
Gut Health Support – Blood Sugar Management

Storage & Reheating:
Best enjoyed fresh. If needed, store in a sealed container in the refrigerator for up to 12 hours. Stir before serving.

Budget-Friendly Notes:
Frozen berries are a more cost-effective alternative to fresh, especially when out of season.
Serving Size: 1 bowl (about 300ml)

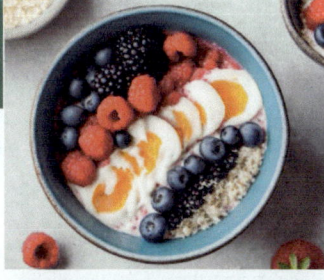

Nutrition Information: (Per Serving)
- Calories: 250 kcal
- Protein: 5g
- Carbohydrates: 30g
- Fiber: 9g
- Sugars: 12g
- Fat: 15g

3. Tropical Detox Smoothie

Yield: 1 serving *Prep Time: 5 minutes* *Cooking Time: None* *Total Time: 5 minutes* *Difficulty Level: Easy*

Description: This refreshing Tropical Detox Smoothie combines the tropical flavors of mango, papaya, and banana with a hint of mint and lime. Packed with nutrients, it supports gut health, detoxification, and overall well-being. Perfect for a light breakfast or snack.

Ingredients:
- 60g / ½ cup mango chunks (fresh or frozen)
- 60g / ½ cup papaya chunks (fresh or frozen)
- 50g / ½ banana
- 15ml / 1 tablespoon coconut milk
- 15ml / 1 tablespoon lime juice
- 1 tablespoon fresh mint leaves (about 6-8 leaves)
- 120ml / ½ cup water or coconut water
- 1 tablespoon hydrolyzed collagen powder (optional)

Instructions:
1. Place all ingredients into a blender.
2. Blend until smooth and creamy.
3. Pour into a glass, garnish with a mint leaf if desired, and enjoy.

Dietary Main Goals:
Weight Loss – Gut Health Support – Blood Sugar Management

Storage & Reheating:
Best consumed immediately after preparation for maximum freshness and nutrient retention.
If storing, place in an airtight container and refrigerate for up to 24 hours. Stir or shake before consuming.

Budget-Friendly Notes:
Use frozen mango and papaya for a cost-effective option, especially when out of season.
Buying in bulk and freezing portions of fruit can reduce costs over time.
Serving Size: 1 smoothie (approximately 300ml)

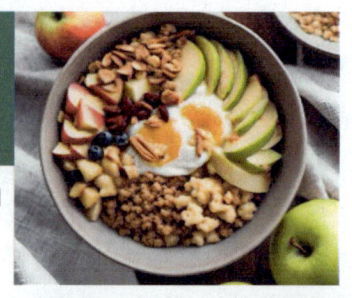

Nutrition Information: (Per Serving)
- Calories: 180 kcal
- Protein: 6g
- Carbohydrates: 34g
- Fiber: 5g
- Sugars: 20g
- Fat: 4g

4. Apple-Cinnamon Cauliflower Breakfast Bowl

Yield: 1 serving *Prep Time: 5 minutes* *Cooking Time: 7 minutes* *Total Time: 12 minutes* *Difficulty Level: Moderate*

Description: This Carrot Cake Smoothie tastes like a delicious slice of cake in a glass, but it's packed with healthy ingredients. A perfect way to sneak in some veggies first thing in the morning!

Ingredients:
- 120g / 1 cup cauliflower rice (fresh or frozen)
- 60g / ½ apple, diced
- 60ml / ¼ cup coconut milk
- 15g / 1 tablespoon raisins
- 7g / 1 tablespoon shredded coconut
- 1g / 1 teaspoon cinnamon
- 5ml / 1 teaspoon vanilla extract
- 5ml / 1 teaspoon honey or maple syrup (optional)
- A pinch of sea salt

Instructions:
1. Combine cauliflower rice, coconut milk, cinnamon, vanilla extract, and sea salt in a small pot.
2. Cook over medium heat, stirring occasionally, until cauliflower is tender and the mixture is creamy (about 5-7 minutes).
3. Remove from heat and stir in diced apple and raisins.
4. If desired, top with shredded coconut and a drizzle of honey or maple syrup.

Dietary Main Goals:
Gut Health Support – Weight Loss

Storage & Reheating:
Can be stored in an airtight container in the refrigerator for up to 2 days. Reheat in a microwave or on the stovetop until warm.

Budget-Friendly Notes:
Cauliflower rice can be made at home using fresh cauliflower, which may be more cost-effective than buying pre-made rice.
Use seasonal apples to save on costs.
Serving Size: 1 bowl

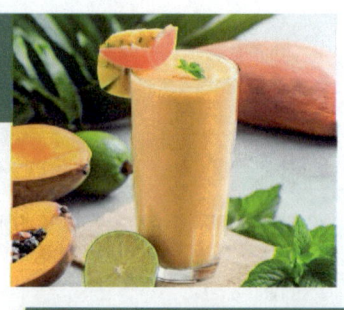

Nutrition Information: (Per Serving)
- Calories: 210 kcal
- Protein: 3g
- Carbohydrates: 28g
- Fiber: 6g
- Sugars: 15g
- Fat: 10g

5. Carrot Cake Smoothie

Yield: 1 serving | Prep Time: 5 minutes | Cooking Time: None | Total Time: 5 minutes | Difficulty Level: Easy

Description: This Carrot Cake Smoothie tastes like a delicious slice of cake in a glass, but it's packed with healthy ingredients. A perfect way to sneak in some veggies first thing in the morning!

Ingredients:
- 120ml / ½ cup carrot juice
- 120ml / ½ cup coconut milk
- 50g / ½ banana
- 30g / ¼ cup shredded carrots
- 1g / ½ teaspoon ground cinnamon
- 1g / ¼ teaspoon ground ginger
- 1g / ¼ teaspoon ground turmeric
- 7g / 1 tablespoon unsweetened coconut flakes
- 1 tablespoon hydrolyzed collagen powder (optional)
- Ice cubes (optional for thicker texture)

Instructions:
1. Add all ingredients to a blender.
2. Blend until smooth and creamy.
3. If desired, pour into a glass, top with additional coconut flakes, and serve immediately.

Dietary Main Goals:
Gut Health Support

Storage & Reheating:
Best consumed immediately. If needed, store in the refrigerator for up to 24 hours. Shake or stir well before consuming.

Budget-Friendly Notes:
Use fresh carrots to make your own carrot juice for a budget-friendly option. Buy coconut flakes in bulk for savings over time.
Serving Size: 1 smoothie (approximately 300ml)

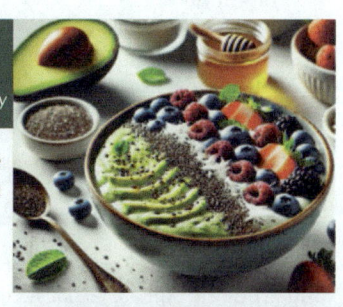

Nutrition Information: (Per Serving)
- Calories: 190 kcal
- Protein: 6g
- Carbohydrates: 25g
- Fiber: 4g
- Sugars: 10g
- Fat: 10g

6. Creamy Avocado and Berry Breakfast Bowl

Yield: 1 serving | Prep Time: 10 minutes | Cooking Time: None | Total Time: 10 minutes | Difficulty Level: Easy

Description: This vibrant Creamy Avocado and Berry Breakfast Bowl is a delightful way to start the day. Combining healthy fats from avocado with nutrient-rich berries, it's a nutritious, filling option for any morning.

Ingredients:
- ½ avocado, mashed (70g)
- 70g / ½ cup mixed berries (blueberries, strawberries)
- 60ml / ¼ cup coconut milk
- 10g / 1 tablespoon chia seeds
- 7g / 1 tablespoon coconut flakes
- 5ml / 1 teaspoon lemon juice
- 5ml / 1 teaspoon honey (optional)
- Fresh mint leaves for garnish (optional)

Instructions:
1. In a bowl, mix mashed avocado, coconut milk, lemon juice, and chia seeds until well combined.
2. Let the mixture sit for 10 minutes to allow the chia seeds to absorb the liquid and thicken.
3. Top with mixed berries and coconut flakes.
4. Drizzle with honey if desired, and garnish with fresh mint leaves.
5. Serve chilled.

Dietary Main Goals:
Gut Health Support – Weight Loss

Storage & Reheating:
Best consumed fresh, but you can refrigerate for up to 24 hours in an airtight container. Stir well before serving.

Budget-Friendly Notes:
Use fresh carrots to make your own carrot juice for a budget-friendly option. Buy coconut flakes in bulk for savings over time.
Serving Size: 1 smoothie (approximately 300ml)

Nutrition Information: (Per Serving)
- Calories: 240 kcal
- Protein: 4g
- Carbohydrates: 22g
- Fiber: 8g
- Sugars: 10g
- Fat: 18g

7. Sweet Potato and Kale Breakfast Hash

Yield: 1 serving   Prep Time: 10 minutes   Cooking Time: 15 minutes   Total Time: 25 minutes
Difficulty Level: Easy

Description: A hearty and nutrient-packed breakfast hash combining sweet potatoes, kale, and vegetables. This dish supports gut health and provides a filling start to the day.

Ingredients:
- 100g / ½ medium sweet potato, peeled and diced
- 60g / ½ cup kale, chopped
- 40g / ¼ onion, diced
- 40g / ¼ bell pepper, diced
- 15ml / 1 tablespoon olive oil
- 1g / ¼ teaspoon turmeric
- Salt and pepper to taste

Instructions:
1. Prepare ingredients: Peel and dice the sweet potato. Wash and chop the kale. Dice the onion and bell pepper.
2. Heat oil in a medium skillet over medium heat.
3. Add diced sweet potato to the skillet and cook for 5-7 minutes, stirring occasionally, until softened and slightly browned.
4. Stir in diced onion and bell pepper. Season with turmeric, salt, and pepper. Cook for another 5 minutes.
5. Add chopped kale, stir well, and cook for 3-4 minutes until the kale wilts and turns bright green.
6. Serve immediately.

Dietary Main Goals:
Weight Loss – Gut Health Support

Storage & Reheating:
Store in an airtight container in the refrigerator for up to 2 days. Reheat in a skillet or microwave until warm.

Budget-Friendly Notes:
Buy sweet potatoes and kale in bulk for cost savings. Frozen kale is a cheaper alternative and works well in this recipe.
Serving Size: 1 bowl

Nutrition Information: (Per Serving)
- Calories: 180 kcal
- Protein: 3g
- Carbohydrates: 25g
- Fiber: 6g
- Sugars: 7g
- Fat: 9g

8. Plantain and Spinach Scramble

Yield: 1 serving   Prep Time: 5 minutes   Cooking Time: 8 minutes   Total Time: 25 minutes
Difficulty Level: Easy

Description: A tropical twist on a traditional scramble, this dish features crispy plantains, spinach, and aromatic spices. Great for gut health and a quick AIP-friendly breakfast

Ingredients:
- 60g / ½ ripe plantain, peeled and diced
- 60g / ½ cup spinach, chopped
- 30ml / 2 tablespoons coconut oil
- 40g / ¼ onion, diced
- 1g / ¼ teaspoon garlic powder
- Salt to taste

Instructions:
1. Peel and dice the plantain into small cubes. Chop the spinach and dice the onion.
2. Heat coconut oil in a medium skillet over medium heat.
3. Add diced plantain to the skillet and cook for 3-4 minutes, stirring occasionally until golden and crispy.
4. Stir in the diced onion and cook for 2 minutes until softened.
5. Add chopped spinach, garlic powder, and salt. Stir and cook for 2-3 minutes until spinach wilts.
6. Serve warm.

Dietary Main Goals:
Gut Health Support – Weight Loss

Storage & Reheating:
Best eaten immediately, but can be stored for up to 1 day in the refrigerator. Reheat in a skillet over medium heat until warm.

Budget-Friendly Notes:
Use frozen spinach for a more economical option. Plantains are often affordable and can be bought in bulk.
Serving Size: 1 scramble

Nutrition Information: (Per Serving)
- Calories: 230 kcal
- Protein: 2g
- Carbohydrates: 26g
- Fiber: 3g
- Sugars: 12g
- Fat: 14g

9. AIP Blueberry Coconut Smoothie

Yield: 1 serving Prep Time: 5 minutes Cooking Time: None Total Time: 5 minutes Difficulty Level: Easy

Description: This refreshing AIP Blueberry Coconut Smoothie is rich in antioxidants and healthy fats, making it a perfect quick breakfast or snack option for supporting gut health.

Ingredients:
- 70g / ½ cup blueberries (fresh or frozen)
- 120ml / ½ cup coconut milk
- 120ml / ½ cup water
- 10g / 1 tablespoon chia seeds
- 15ml / 1 tablespoon coconut oil
- 5ml / 1 teaspoon honey (optional)

Instructions:
1. Combine all ingredients in a blender.
2. Blend until smooth.
3. Pour into a glass and serve immediately.

Dietary Main Goals:
Gut Health Support – Weight Loss

Storage & Reheating:
Best consumed immediately but can be stored for up to 24 hours in a refrigerator. Shake or stir before consuming.

Budget-Friendly Notes:
Use frozen blueberries for a cost-saving option. Chia seeds can be bought in bulk for long-term use.
Serving Size: 1 smoothie (approximately 300ml)

Nutrition Information: (Per Serving)
- Calories: 180 kcal
- Protein: 3g
- Carbohydrates: 18g
- Fiber: 6g
- Sugars: 8g
- Fat: 14g

---

10. Baked Apple Cinnamon Breakfast Bowl

Yield: 1 serving Prep Time: 10 minutes Cooking Time: 20 minutes Total Time: 30 minutes
Difficulty Level: Moderate

Description: A tropical twist on a traditional scramble, this dish features crispy plantains, spinach, and aromatic spices. Great for gut health and a quick AIP-friendly breakfast.

Ingredients:
- medium apple, diced (150g / 1 apple)
- 60ml / ¼ cup unsweetened applesauce
- 15g / 1 tablespoon coconut flour
- 15g / 1 tablespoon raisins
- 2g / ½ teaspoon cinnamon
- 5ml / 1 teaspoon coconut oil

Instructions:
1. Preheat oven to 350°F (175°C).
2. Mix diced apple, applesauce, coconut flour, raisins, and cinnamon in a bowl.
3. Grease a small baking dish with coconut oil and pour in the mixture.
4. Bake for 20 minutes until the apples are tender.
5. Serve warm.

Dietary Main Goals:
Blood Sugar Management – Gut Health Support

Storage & Reheating:
Can be stored in the refrigerator for up to 2 days. Reheat in the microwave or oven until warm.

Budget-Friendly Notes:
Use frozen blueberries for a cost-saving option. Chia seeds can be bought in bulk for long-term use.
Serving Size: 1 smoothie (approximately 300ml)

Nutrition Information: (Per Serving)
- Calories: 220 kcal
- Protein: 2g
- Carbohydrates: 38g
- Fiber: 6g
- Sugars: 25g
- Fat: 8g

11. Carrot and Ginger Smoothie Bowl

Yield: 1 serving | Prep Time: 5 minutes | Cooking Time: None | Total Time: 5 minutes | Difficulty Level: Easy

Description: A refreshing and zesty smoothie bowl packed with the anti-inflammatory benefits of ginger and carrots. This bowl is perfect for gut health and a boost of morning energy.

Ingredients:
- 120ml / ½ cup carrot juice
- ½ frozen banana
- 60ml / ¼ cup coconut milk
- 15g / 1 tablespoon fresh ginger, grated
- 15g / 1 tablespoon collagen peptides (optional)
- 7g / 1 tablespoon coconut flakes

Instructions:
1. Blend carrot juice, banana, coconut milk, ginger, and collagen until smooth.
2. Pour into a bowl and top with coconut flakes.
3. Serve chilled.

Dietary Main Goals:
Gut Health Support – Weight Loss

Storage & Reheating:
Best served fresh. Can be stored in the refrigerator for up to 24 hours. Stir before serving.

Budget-Friendly Notes:
Frozen bananas are a budget-friendly alternative to fresh.
Serving Size: 1 smoothie bowl (about 350ml)

Nutrition Information: (Per Serving)
- Calories: 160 kcal
- Protein: 6g
- Carbohydrates: 24g
- Fiber: 4g
- Sugars: 12g
- Fat: 6g

---

12. Savory Cauliflower and Spinach Breakfast Bowl

Yield: 1 serving | Prep Time: 5 minutes | Cooking Time: 10 minutes | Total Time: 15 minutes | Difficulty Level: Easy

Description: A savory and nutrient-dense breakfast bowl featuring cauliflower rice, spinach, and mushrooms. This dish is great for promoting gut health and inflammation reduction.

Ingredients:
- 120g / ½ cup cauliflower rice
- 60g / ¼ cup spinach, chopped
- 30ml / 2 tablespoons olive oil
- 15g / ⅛ cup mushrooms, sliced
- 1g / ¼ teaspoon turmeric
- Salt and pepper to taste

Instructions:
1. **Prepare ingredients:** Finely chop the spinach, slice the mushrooms, and measure the cauliflower rice.
2. Heat olive oil in a medium skillet over medium heat.
3. Add cauliflower rice and sauté for 4-5 minutes, stirring occasionally until tender and slightly golden.
4. Add spinach, mushrooms, turmeric, salt, and pepper. Stir everything together and cook for another 3-5 minutes until spinach wilts and mushrooms are soft.
5. Serve hot.

Dietary Main Goals:
Gut Health Support – Weight Loss

Storage & Reheating:
Store in an airtight container in the refrigerator for up to 2 days. Reheat in a skillet or microwave until warm.

Budget-Friendly Notes:
Use frozen spinach to reduce costs.
Serving Size: 1 bowl

Nutrition Information: (Per Serving)
- Calories: 150 kcal
- Protein: 2g
- Carbohydrates: 6g
- Fiber: 3g
- Sugars: 2g
- Fat: 12g

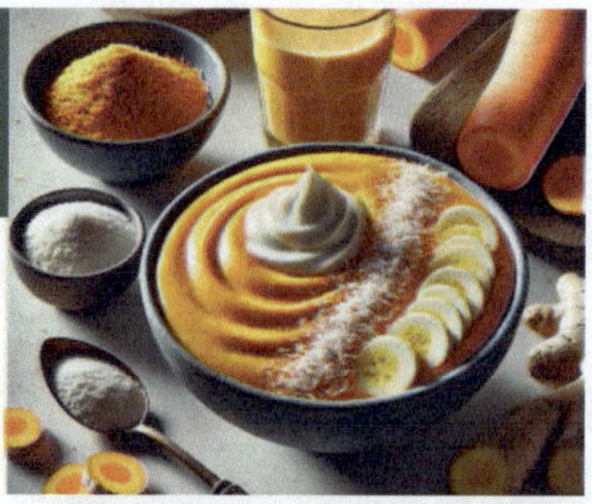

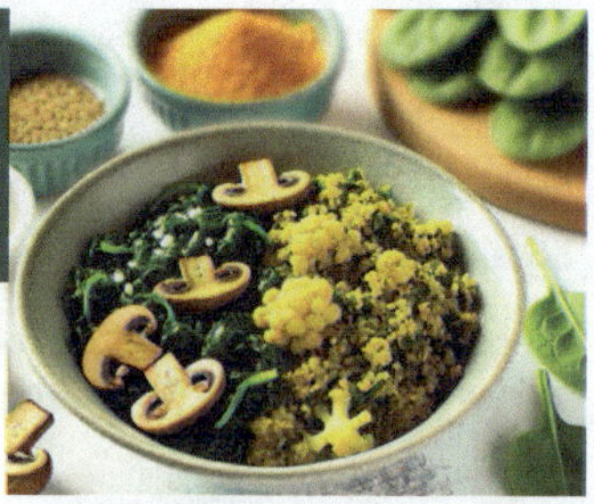

13. AIP Sweet Potato Pancakes

Yield: 1 serving   Prep Time: 10 minutes   Cooking Time: 10 minutes   Total Time: 20 minutes
Difficulty Level: Easy

Description: These fluffy and nutrient-dense sweet potato pancakes are a delicious AIP-friendly breakfast option, perfect for a comforting morning meal.

Ingredients:
- 120g / ½ cup mashed sweet potatoes
- 7g / 1 tablespoon coconut flour
- 15ml / 1 tablespoon coconut milk
- 0.5g / ⅛ teaspoon cinnamon
- 7g / ½ tablespoon coconut oil

Nutrition Information: (Per Serving)
- Calories: 180 kcal
- Protein: 2g
- Carbohydrates: 20g
- Fiber: 4g
- Sugars: 6g
- Fat: 10g

Instructions:
1. Ensure the sweet potatoes are fully cooked and mashed smoothly. Combine mashed sweet potatoes, coconut flour, coconut milk, and cinnamon in a medium bowl. Stir until smooth.
2. Heat coconut oil over medium heat in a skillet.
3. Form small pancakes from the batter and drop onto the hot skillet. Cook for 3 minutes on each side until golden.
4. Serve warm.

Dietary Main Goals:
Weight Loss – Gut Health Support

Storage & Reheating:
Store in an airtight container in the refrigerator for up to 2 days. Reheat in a skillet or microwave.

Budget-Friendly Notes:
Use leftover mashed sweet potatoes to save time and money.
Serving Size: 1 bowl

14. Coconut Plantain Porridge

Yield: 1 serving   Prep Time: 5 minutes   Cooking Time: 7 minutes   Total Time: 12 minutes
Difficulty Level: Easy

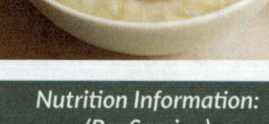

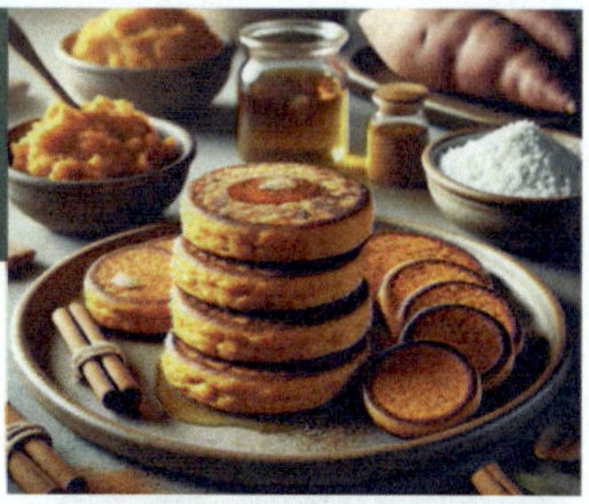

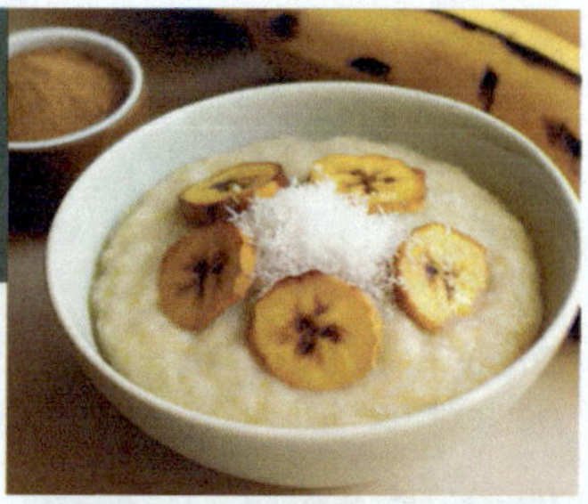

Description: This warm and creamy porridge made from plantains and coconut milk is a satisfying and nutritious AIP-friendly breakfast option that supports gut health.

Ingredients:
- 1 ripe plantain, sliced
- 120ml / ½ cup coconut milk
- 60ml / ¼ cup water
- 7g / 1 tablespoon shredded coconut
- 2g / ½ teaspoon cinnamon
- 5ml / 1 teaspoon honey (optional)

Nutrition Information: (Per Serving)
- Calories: 250 kcal
- Protein: 2g
- Carbohydrates: 45g
- Fiber: 5g
- Sugars: 12g
- Fat: 10g

Instructions:
1. Blend plantain, coconut milk, and water until smooth.
2. Pour into a saucepan and cook over medium heat for 5-7 minutes, stirring frequently until thickened.
3. Pour into a bowl, top with shredded coconut and cinnamon, and drizzle with honey if desired.
4. Serve warm.

Dietary Main Goals:
Gut Health Support – Blood Sugar Management

Storage & Reheating:
Best enjoyed fresh but can be stored in the fridge for up to 24 hours. Reheat on the stovetop or microwave.

Budget-Friendly Notes:
Use ripe plantains, which are often inexpensive, and buy coconut milk in bulk for cost savings.
Serving Size: 1 bowl

15. Zucchini Breakfast Hash with Ground Turkey

Yield: 2 servings Prep Time: 10 minutes Cooking Time: 12 minutes Total Time: 22 minutes
Difficulty Level: Easy

Description: A hearty and savory breakfast hash combining ground turkey, zucchini, and aromatic spices for a protein-packed start to the day.

Ingredients:
- 1 zucchini, diced
- 225g / ½ lb ground turkey
- 60g / ½ onion, diced
- 30ml / 2 tablespoons olive oil
- 1g / ¼ teaspoon garlic powder
- Salt and pepper to taste

Instructions:
1. Heat olive oil in a skillet over medium heat.
2. Add onion and ground turkey, cooking until turkey is browned (5-7 minutes).
3. Add zucchini, garlic powder, salt, and pepper. Cook for another 5 minutes until tender.
4. Serve hot.

Dietary Main Goals:
Muscle Building – Weight Loss

Storage & Reheating:
BStore leftovers in an airtight container in the refrigerator for up to 2 days. Reheat in a skillet or microwave.

Budget-Friendly Notes:
Ground turkey and zucchini are affordable protein and vegetable options, making this dish budget-friendly.
Serving Size: 1 bowl (serves 2)

Nutrition Information: (Per Serving)
- Calories: 300 kcal
- Protein: 25g
- Carbohydrates: 10g
- Fiber: 2g
- Sugars: 4g
- Fat: 18g

---

16. AIP Apple Cinnamon Smoothie

Yield: 1 serving Prep Time: 5 minutes Cooking Time: None Total Time: 5 minutes
Difficulty Level: Easy

Description: A sweet and satisfying smoothie made with fresh apples, cinnamon, and coconut milk, perfect for a quick, nutrient-rich breakfast or snack.

Ingredients:
- 1 apple, peeled and chopped
- 120ml / ½ cup coconut milk
- 120ml / ½ cup water
- 15g / 1 tablespoon chia seeds
- 2g / ½ teaspoon cinnamon
- 5ml / 1 teaspoon honey (optional)

Instructions:
1. Blend all ingredients until smooth.
2. Pour into a glass and serve immediately.

Dietary Main Goals:
Blood Sugar Management – Gut Health Support

Storage & Reheating:
Best served fresh. If storing, refrigerate for up to 24 hours and stir before serving.

Budget-Friendly Notes:
Apples and chia seeds are affordable, making this recipe budget-friendly.
Serving Size: 1 smoothie (about 300ml)

Nutrition Information: (Per Serving)
- Calories: 180 kcal
- Protein: 2g
- Carbohydrates: 30g
- Fiber: 5g
- Sugars: 18g
- Fat: 7g

17. Collard Greens and Bacon Breakfast Wrap

Yield: 1 serving Prep Time: 5 minutes Cooking Time: 10 minutes Total Time: 15 minutes
Difficulty Level: Easy

Description: A simple yet flavorful breakfast wrap made with crispy AIP-compliant bacon, avocado, and collard greens for a nutrient-packed and satisfying start to the day.

Ingredients:
- 4 large collard green leaves
- 4 slices AIP-compliant bacon
- ½ avocado, sliced
- 60g / ½ cup shredded carrots
- 15ml / 1 tablespoon olive oil

Instructions:
1. Cook bacon until crispy and set aside.
2. Lightly steam collard green leaves to soften.
3. Place bacon, avocado, and carrots in the center of each leaf.
4. Roll tightly and secure with toothpicks.
5. Serve immediately.

Dietary Main Goals:
Gut Health Support – Weight Loss

Storage & Reheating:
Best served fresh. Can be stored for up to 12 hours in the refrigerator.

Budget-Friendly Notes:
Use affordable AIP-compliant bacon and collard greens for a budget-friendly meal.
Serving Size: 1 wrap (serves 2)

Nutrition Information: (Per Serving)
- Calories: 220 kcal
- Protein: 10g
- Carbohydrates: 12g
- Fiber: 5g
- Sugars: 2g
- Fat: 16g

---

18. AIP Pumpkin Breakfast Porridge

Yield: 1 serving Prep Time: 5 minutes Cooking Time: 7 minutes Total Time: 12 minutes
Difficulty Level: Easy

Description: A warm and comforting breakfast porridge made from pumpkin puree and coconut milk, with a touch of cinnamon for a cozy start to the day.

Ingredients:
- 120g / ½ cup pumpkin puree
- 120ml / ½ cup coconut milk
- 120ml / ½ cup water
- 15g / 1 tablespoon coconut flour
- 1g / ¼ teaspoon cinnamon
- 15ml / 1 tablespoon maple syrup (optional)

Instructions:
1. Combine pumpkin puree, coconut milk, water, coconut flour, and cinnamon in a saucepan.
2. Cook over medium heat, stirring constantly, until thickened (5-7 minutes).
3. Pour into a bowl and drizzle with maple syrup if desired.
4. Serve warm.

Dietary Main Goals:
Gut Health Support – Blood Sugar Management

Storage & Reheating:
Store in an airtight container for up to 24 hours. Reheat on the stovetop or microwave before serving.

Budget-Friendly Notes:
Canned pumpkin puree is an affordable and convenient ingredient.
Serving Size: 1 bowl

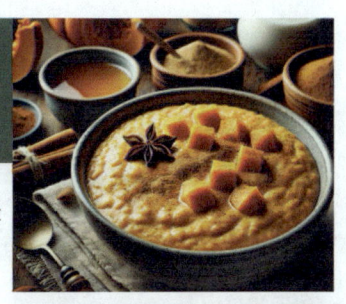

Nutrition Information: (Per Serving)
- Calories: 190 kcal
- Protein: 3g
- Carbohydrates: 24g
- Fiber: 4g
- Sugars: 10g
- Fat: 12g

19. AIP Sweet Potato and Apple Hash

Yield: 2 servings | Prep Time: 10 minutes | Cooking Time: 10 minutes | Total Time: 20 minutes
Difficulty Level: Easy

Description: A flavorful, nutrient-dense hash made with sweet potatoes, apples, and cinnamon. Perfect for a satisfying and nutritious breakfast or side dish.

Ingredients:
- 1 apple, diced
- 60g / ½ onion, diced
- 30ml / 2 tablespoons coconut oil
- 1g / ½ teaspoon cinnamon
- Salt to taste

Instructions:
1. Heat coconut oil in a skillet over medium heat.
2. Add sweet potato and cook for 5 minutes.
3. Add apple, onion, cinnamon, and salt. Cook for another 5 minutes until tender.
4. Serve hot.

Dietary Main Goals:
Blood Sugar Management – Weight Loss

Storage & Reheating:
Store leftovers in an airtight container for up to 24 hours. Reheat in a skillet or microwave before serving.

Budget-Friendly Notes:
Sweet potatoes and apples are affordable and readily available year-round.
Serving Size: 1 bowl (serves 2)

Nutrition Information: (Per Serving)
- Calories: 250 kcal
- Protein: 2g
- Carbohydrates: 38g
- Fiber: 6g
- Sugars: 18g
- Fat: 10g

---

20. Butternut Squash and Sausage Breakfast Bake

Yield: 2 servings | Prep Time: 10 minutes | Cooking Time: 25 minutes | Total Time: 35 minutes
Difficulty Level: Moderate

Description: A delicious and filling breakfast bake featuring butternut squash, AIP-compliant sausage, and spinach, perfect for a hearty morning meal.

Ingredients:
- 240g / 1 cup butternut squash, diced
- 225g / ½ lb AIP-compliant sausage
- 60g / ½ cup spinach, chopped
- 60g / ½ onion, diced
- 30ml / 2 tablespoons olive oil

Instructions:
1. Preheat oven to 375°F (190°C).
2. In a skillet, heat olive oil over medium heat. Cook sausage and onion for 5 minutes until browned.
3. Add butternut squash and spinach, and cook for another 5 minutes.
4. Transfer to a baking dish and bake for 20 minutes.
5. Serve warm.

Dietary Main Goals:
Muscle Building – Gut Health Support

Storage & Reheating:
Store leftovers in an airtight container for up to 2 days. Reheat in the oven or microwave before serving.

Budget-Friendly Notes:
Butternut squash and spinach are affordable, nutritious ingredients. Bulk sausage can be cost-effective.
Serving Size: 1 serving (serves 2)

Nutrition Information: (Per Serving)
- Calories: 320 kcal
- Protein: 18g
- Carbohydrates: 16g
- Fiber: 4g
- Sugars: 4g
- Fat: 22g

21. AIP Banana Coconut Porridge

Yield: 1 serving Prep Time: 5 minutes Cooking Time: 5 minutes Total Time: 10 minutes
Difficulty Level: Easy

Description: A creamy and tropical porridge made with mashed bananas, coconut milk, and a hint of cinnamon. This simple and satisfying breakfast is AIP-friendly and nutrient-dense.

Ingredients:
- 1 ripe banana, mashed
- 60ml / ¼ cup coconut milk
- 15g / 1 tablespoon coconut flour
- 1g / ¼ teaspoon cinnamon
- 7g / 1 tablespoon shredded coconut (optional)
- 2ml / ½ teaspoon vanilla extract
- A pinch of salt

Nutrition Information: (Per Serving)
- Calories: 180 kcal
- Protein: 2g
- Carbohydrates: 24g
- Fiber: 5g
- Sugars: 10g
- Fat: 9g

Instructions:
1. Combine mashed banana, coconut milk, coconut flour, cinnamon, vanilla extract, and a pinch of salt in a small saucepan.
2. Cook over medium heat, stirring constantly, until thickened (about 3-4 minutes).
3. Remove from heat and transfer to a bowl. Sprinkle shredded coconut on top if desired.
4. Serve warm.

Dietary Main Goals:
Gut Health Support – Weight Loss

Storage & Reheating:
Best served fresh, but can be refrigerated for up to 24 hours. Reheat in a saucepan or microwave.

Budget-Friendly Notes:
Bananas and coconut milk are inexpensive, making this a budget-friendly recipe.
Serving Size: 1 bowl

---

22. AIP Apple Cinnamon Breakfast Sausage

Yield: 1-2 serving Prep Time: 10 minutes Cooking Time: 10 minutes Total Time: 20 minutes
Difficulty Level: Easy

Description: This savory breakfast sausage has a touch of sweetness from grated apple and warm spice from cinnamon, making it a flavorful and protein-packed option for an AIP-compliant breakfast.

Ingredients:
- 225g / ½ lb ground pork (or turkey)
- 30g / ¼ cup grated apple
- 1g / ¼ teaspoon cinnamon
- 1g / ¼ teaspoon ground sage
- 15ml / 1 tablespoon coconut oil
- Salt to taste

Nutrition Information: (Per Serving)
- Calories: 250 kcal
- Protein: 17g
- Carbohydrates: 7g
- Fiber: 1g
- Sugars: 4g
- Fat: 18g

Instructions:
1. In a mixing bowl, combine the ground pork, grated apple, cinnamon, ground sage, and salt. Mix well.
2. Form the mixture into small sausage patties.
3. Heat 1 tablespoon of coconut oil in a skillet over medium heat.
4. Cook the patties on each side for 4-5 minutes until golden brown is cooked through.
5. Serve warm.

Dietary Main Goals:
Muscle Building – Gut Health Support

Storage & Reheating:
Store leftovers in an airtight container in the refrigerator for up to 2 days. Reheat in a skillet or microwave before serving.

Budget-Friendly Notes:
Ground pork is typically more affordable than turkey. Apples are a cost-effective way to add natural sweetness.
Serving Size: 1-2 patties (depending on size)

23. Chicken and Avocado Collard Wraps

Yield: 1 serving | Prep Time: 10 minutes | Cooking Time: None | Total Time: 10 minutes | Difficulty Level: Easy

Description: A refreshing and nutrient-packed wrap with shredded chicken, creamy avocado, and crunchy carrots, all wrapped in tender collard greens. A perfect choice for a quick and healthy meal.

Ingredients:
- 2 large collard green leaves
- 100g / ½ cup cooked chicken breast, shredded
- 60g / ½ avocado, sliced
- 30g / ¼ cup shredded carrots
- 30g / 2 tablespoons sauerkraut
- 15ml / 1 tablespoon olive oil
- Salt to taste

Instructions:
1. Lightly steam the collard leaves to soften.
2. Lay a collard leaf flat and layer it with shredded chicken, avocado slices, carrots, and sauerkraut.
3. Drizzle with olive oil and sprinkle with salt.
4. Roll the leaf tightly and secure it with a toothpick.
5. Serve immediately.

Dietary Main Goals:
Gut Health Support – Weight Loss

Storage & Reheating:
Best served fresh. Can be stored in the refrigerator for up to 12 hours.

Budget-Friendly Notes:
Use leftover chicken for cost efficiency.
Serving Size: 1 wrap

Nutrition Information: (Per Serving)
- Calories: 280 kcal
- Protein: 20g
- Carbohydrates: 14g
- Fiber: 6g
- Sugars: 2g
- Fat: 18g

---

24. Hearty Kale and Sweet Potato Salad with Ground Beef

Yield: 2 servings | Prep Time: 10 minutes | Cooking Time: 15 minutes | Total Time: 25 minutes | Difficulty Level: Easy

Description: This hearty salad combines nutritious kale, sweet potatoes, and ground beef for a delicious, protein-packed meal that can be served warm or cold.

Ingredients:
- 115g / ¼ lb ground beef (grass-fed)
- 60g / 1 cup kale, chopped
- 100g / ½ medium sweet potato, diced
- 15ml / 1 tablespoon olive oil
- 5ml / 1 teaspoon apple cider vinegar
- 5ml / 1 teaspoon coconut aminos
- 1g / ⅛ teaspoon garlic powder
- Salt and pepper to taste

Instructions:
1. In a skillet, cook the ground beef until browned. Set aside.
2. In the same skillet, sauté sweet potatoes in 1 tablespoon of olive oil for about 8 minutes until soft.
3. Massage the kale in a bowl with olive oil and apple cider vinegar.
4. Combine kale, sweet potatoes, and ground beef. Drizzle with coconut aminos and garlic powder.
5. Serve warm or cold.

Dietary Main Goals:
Muscle Building – Blood Sugar Management

Storage & Reheating:
Can be refrigerated for up to 24 hours. Reheat in a skillet or enjoy cold.

Budget-Friendly Notes:
Ground beef and kale are cost-effective and filling ingredients.
Serving Size: 1 bowl

Nutrition Information: (Per Serving)
- Calories: 450 kcal
- Protein: 30g
- Carbohydrates: 20g
- Fiber: 6g
- Sugars: 4g
- Fat: 28g

25. AIP Salmon and Spinach Wrap

Yield: 1 serving Prep Time: 5 minutes Cooking Time: None Total Time: 5 minutes Difficulty Level: Easy

Description: A light and flavorful wrap made with wild-caught salmon, creamy avocado, and fresh spinach, all wrapped in crisp romaine leaves. Perfect for a quick, healthy lunch.

Ingredients:
- 1 large romaine lettuce leaf
- 75g / ½ can wild-caught salmon, drained
- 60g / ½ avocado, mashed
- 30g / ¼ cup fresh spinach, chopped
- 15ml / 1 tablespoon olive oil
- 15ml / 1 tablespoon lemon juice
- Salt to taste

Instructions:
1. In a bowl, mix salmon, mashed avocado, spinach, olive oil, lemon juice, and salt.
2. Spoon the mixture onto the romaine leaf.
3. Roll the leaf into a wrap and serve immediately.

Dietary Main Goals:
Gut Health Support – Weight Loss

Storage & Reheating:
Best served fresh, but can be stored in the fridge for up to 12 hours

Budget-Friendly Notes:
Canned salmon is an affordable protein source.
Serving Size: 1 wrap

Nutrition Information: (Per Serving)
- Calories: 220 kcal
- Protein: 18g
- Carbohydrates: 8g
- Fiber: 4g
- Sugars: 1g
- Fat: 15g

---

26. Gut-Healing Bone Broth Chicken Soup

Yield: 1 serving Prep Time: 10 minutes Cooking Time: 20 minutes Total Time: 30 minutes Difficulty Level: Moderate

Description: A nutrient-rich, gut-healing soup featuring bone broth, shredded chicken, and a variety of vegetables. This comforting soup supports digestion and immunity.

Ingredients:
- 240ml / 1 cup bone broth
- 75g / ⅓ cup cooked chicken breast, shredded
- 60g / ¼ cup carrots, sliced
- 60g / ¼ cup celery, sliced
- 30g / ¼ cup kale, chopped
- 5ml / 1 teaspoon coconut oil
- 2g / ½ teaspoon fresh ginger, grated
- Salt to taste

Instructions:
1. Heat coconut oil in a small pot over medium heat.
2. Add carrots, celery, and ginger; sauté for 5 minutes.
3. Pour in bone broth and bring to a boil. Reduce heat and simmer for 10 minutes.
4. Add shredded chicken and kale, cooking for an additional 5 minutes.
5. Serve hot.

Dietary Main Goals:
Gut Health Support – Weight Loss

Storage & Reheating:
Store in the refrigerator for up to 2 days. Reheat on the stovetop or in the microwave.

Budget-Friendly Notes:
Homemade bone broth from leftover bones can save costs.
Serving Size: 1 bowl

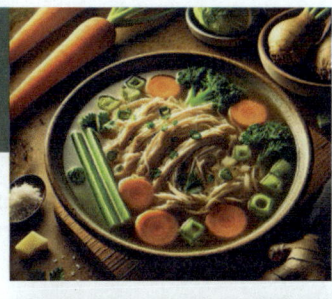

Nutrition Information: (Per Serving)
- Calories: 180 kcal
- Protein: 16g
- Carbohydrates: 10g
- Fiber: 3g
- Sugars: 3g
- Fat: 9g

27. Beef and Cauliflower Rice Stir-Fry

Yield: 1 serving Prep Time: 10 minutes Cooking Time: 15 minutes Total Time: 25 minutes
Difficulty Level: Easy

Description: A quick and flavorful stir-fry combining ground beef, cauliflower rice, and vegetables. It's packed with protein and nutrients, making it a perfect weeknight meal.

Ingredients:
- 120g / 1 cup cauliflower rice
- 60g / ¼ cup broccoli florets
- 60g / ¼ cup carrots, sliced
- 30ml / 2 tablespoons coconut aminos
- 15ml / 1 tablespoon olive oil
- 2.5g / ½ teaspoon ginger powder
- Salt to taste

Instructions:
1. Heat olive oil in a skillet over medium heat.
2. Cook ground beef until browned, then remove and set aside.
3. In the same skillet, sauté broccoli, carrots, and cauliflower rice for 5-7 minutes until tender.
4. Return the ground beef to the skillet, stir in coconut aminos, ginger powder, and salt.

Dietary Main Goals:
Muscle Building – Gut Health Support

Storage & Reheating:
Muscle Building – Gut Health Support

Budget-Friendly Notes:
Cauliflower rice can be homemade from fresh cauliflower to reduce costs.
Serving Size: 1 bowl

Nutrition Information: (Per Serving)
- Calories: 320 kcal
- Protein: 25g
- Carbohydrates: 12g
- Fiber: 4g
- Sugars: 3g
- Fat: 20g

28. Herbed Turkey and Butternut Squash Salad

Yield: 1 serving Prep Time: 10 minutes Cooking Time: 20 minutes Total Time: 30 minutes
Difficulty Level: Easy

Description: A vibrant and hearty salad featuring shredded turkey and roasted butternut squash, served over a bed of mixed greens and drizzled with a simple herb dressing.

Ingredients:
- 100g / ½ cup cooked turkey breast, shredded
- 120g / 1 cup butternut squash, roasted and diced
- 60g / 1 cup mixed greens (spinach, arugula)
- 30ml / 2 tablespoons olive oil
- 10ml / 2 teaspoons apple cider vinegar
- 2g / 1 teaspoon dried rosemary
- Salt and pepper to taste

Instructions:
1. In a bowl, combine turkey, roasted butternut squash, and mixed greens.
2. Whisk together olive oil, apple cider vinegar, rosemary, salt, and pepper.
3. Drizzle the dressing over the salad and toss well.
4. Serve immediately.

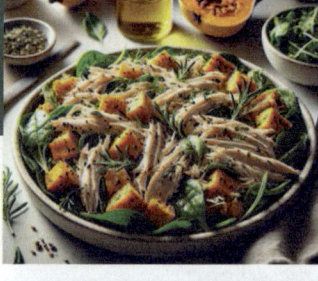

Dietary Main Goals:
Muscle Building – Gut Health Support

Storage & Reheating:
Store in an airtight container for up to 12 hours. Best served fresh.

Budget-Friendly Notes:
Roasting your own butternut squash from fresh is more affordable than buying pre-cut.
Serving Size: 1 bowl

Nutrition Information: (Per Serving)
- Calories: 300 kcal
- Protein: 28g
- Carbohydrates: 20g
- Fiber: 5g
- Sugars: 6g
- Fat: 15g

29. Ginger-Turmeric Chicken and Cabbage Soup

Yield: 1 serving Prep Time: 10 minutes Cooking Time: 20 minutes Total Time: 30 minutes
Difficulty Level: Moderate

Description: A warming and anti-inflammatory soup featuring chicken, cabbage, and the healing properties of ginger and turmeric. Perfect for gut health support.

Ingredients:
- 115g / ¼ lb chicken thighs, cubed
- 240ml / 1 cup chicken bone broth
- 60g / ½ cup green cabbage, shredded
- 60g / ¼ cup carrots, diced
- 5g / 1 tablespoon fresh ginger, minced
- 1g / ½ teaspoon turmeric
- 5ml / 1 teaspoon coconut oil
- Salt to taste

Instructions:
1. Heat coconut oil in a pot over medium heat.
2. Add chicken thighs and cook until browned.
3. Add ginger, turmeric, carrots, and cabbage. Cook for 5 minutes.
4. Pour in bone broth and bring to a boil. Simmer for 15 minutes.
5. Serve hot.

Dietary Main Goals:
Gut Health Support – Weight Loss

Storage & Reheating:
Store in an airtight container for up to 2 days. Reheat on the stovetop or microwave before serving.

Budget-Friendly Notes:
Using chicken thighs instead of breasts makes this dish more affordable.
Serving Size: 1 bowl

Nutrition Information: (Per Serving)
- Calories: 250 kcal
- Protein: 22g
- Carbohydrates: 10g
- Fiber: 3g
- Sugars: 3g
- Fat: 15g

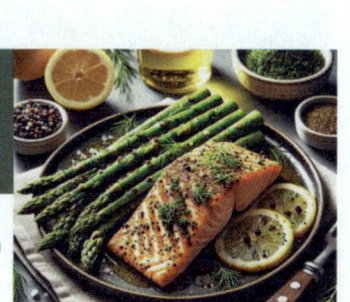

---

30. Lemon Herb Salmon with Asparagus

Yield: 1 serving Prep Time: 5 minutes Cooking Time: 20 minutes Total Time: 25 minutes
Difficulty Level: Easy

Description: A light and flavorful dish of baked salmon fillets with tender asparagus, seasoned with fresh lemon and herbs. This meal is quick, nutritious, and ideal for muscle building.

Ingredients:
- 1 salmon fillet (115g / 4 oz, wild-caught)
- 100g / ½ bunch asparagus, trimmed
- 15ml / 1 tablespoon olive oil
- 5ml / 1 teaspoon lemon juice
- 1g / ½ teaspoon dried dill
- Salt and pepper to taste

Instructions:
1. Preheat oven to 375°F (190°C).
2. Place salmon and asparagus on a baking sheet. Drizzle with olive oil, lemon juice, dill, salt, and pepper.
3. Bake for 15-20 minutes until salmon is cooked through.
4. Serve hot.

Dietary Main Goals:
Muscle Building – Gut Health Support

Storage & Reheating:
Can be refrigerated for up to 24 hours. Reheat in the oven or microwave

Budget-Friendly Notes:
Using frozen salmon fillets can help reduce costs.
Serving Size: 1 fillet

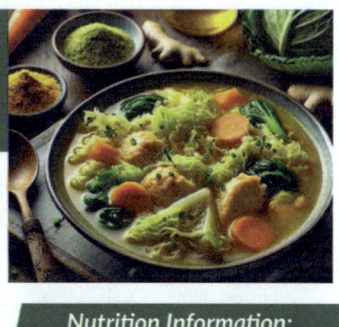

Nutrition Information: (Per Serving)
- Calories: 350 kcal
- Protein: 28g
- Carbohydrates: 8g
- Fiber: 4g
- Sugars: 2g
- Fat: 24g

31. Sweet Potato and Beef Stew

Yield: 1 serving Prep Time: 10 minutes Cooking Time: 35 minutes Total Time: 45 minutes
Difficulty Level: Moderate

Description: A hearty and comforting stew with tender beef, sweet potatoes, and carrots simmered in rich bone broth, perfect for a filling and nourishing meal.

Ingredients:
- 115g / ¼ lb grass-fed beef stew meat
- 120g / 1 cup sweet potatoes, diced
- 60g / ½ cup carrots, sliced
- 240ml / 1 cup beef bone broth
- 60g / ½ onion, diced
- 15ml / 1 tablespoon olive oil
- 1g / 1 teaspoon dried thyme
- Salt and pepper to taste

Instructions:
1. Heat olive oil in a large pot over medium heat.
2. Brown beef stew meat, then remove and set aside.
3. Add onion, carrots, and sweet potatoes to the pot. Cook for 5 minutes.
4. Return beef to the pot, and add bone broth, thyme, salt, and pepper.
5. Simmer for 30 minutes until beef is tender.
6. Serve hot.

Dietary Main Goals:
Muscle Building – Gut Health Support

Storage & Reheating:
Store in an airtight container for up to 2 days in the refrigerator. Reheat on the stovetop or microwave.

Budget-Friendly Notes:
Opt for buying beef stew meat in bulk for better savings.
Serving Size: 1 bowl

Nutrition Information: (Per Serving)
- Calories: 380 kcal
- Protein: 28g
- Carbohydrates: 22g
- Fiber: 4g
- Sugars: 5g
- Fat: 20g

32. Coconut-crusted chicken with Spinach Salad

Yield: 1 serving Prep Time: 10 minutes Cooking Time: 20 minutes Total Time: 30 minutes
Difficulty Level: Moderate

Description: A delicious and crispy coconut-crusted chicken served over a fresh spinach and carrot salad, making for a light yet filling meal.

Ingredients:
- 115g / 4 oz small pasture-raised chicken breast
- 30g / ¼ cup coconut flakes
- 15g / 2 tablespoons coconut flour
- 30ml / 2 tablespoons coconut oil
- 60g / 2 cups spinach leaves
- 15g / 2 tablespoons shredded carrots
- 30ml / 2 tablespoons olive oil
- 15ml / 1 tablespoon apple cider vinegar
- Salt and pepper to taste

Instructions:
1. Preheat the oven to 375°F (190°C) and line a baking sheet with parchment paper.
2. Pat the chicken breast dry and season lightly with salt and pepper.
3. Dredge the chicken in coconut flour, then press into coconut flakes to coat.
4. Heat 2 tablespoons of coconut oil in a skillet over medium heat. Sear the chicken for 3 minutes on each side until golden.
5. Transfer the chicken to the prepared baking sheet and bake for 12–15 minutes, until the internal temperature reaches 165°F (75°C).
6. While baking, toss spinach and carrots with olive oil, apple cider vinegar, salt, and pepper.
7. Serve the coconut-crusted chicken on top of the spinach salad.

Dietary Main Goals:
Muscle Building – Weight Loss

Storage & Reheating:
Best served fresh, but can be stored in the fridge for up to 24 hours.

Budget-Friendly Notes:
Using pasture-raised chicken for both quality and affordability.
Serving Size: 1 plate

Nutrition Information: (Per Serving)
- Calories: 210 kcal
- Protein: 17g
- Carbohydrates: 6g
- Fiber: 3g
- Sugars: 1.5g
- Fat: 14g

33. Crispy Chicken and Roasted Vegetable Salad

Yield: 1 serving   Prep Time: 10 minutes   Cooking Time: 30 minutes   Total Time: 40 minutes
Difficulty Level: Moderate

Description: Crispy pan-seared chicken thighs served over a bed of mixed greens with roasted Brussels sprouts and butternut squash.

Ingredients:
- 115g / 2 chicken thighs (pasture-raised)
- 120g / 1 cup Brussels sprouts, halved
- 120g / 1 cup butternut squash, diced
- 60g / 2 cups mixed greens (spinach, arugula)
- 45ml / 3 tablespoons olive oil
- 15ml / 1 tablespoon apple cider vinegar
- 1g / ½ teaspoon garlic powder
- Salt and pepper to taste

Instructions:
1. Preheat oven to 375°F (190°C). Toss Brussels sprouts and butternut squash in 1 tablespoon of olive oil, salt, and pepper. Roast for 20 minutes.
2. Season chicken thighs with salt, pepper, and garlic powder. Pan-sear in 1 tablespoon of olive oil over medium heat until crispy and cooked through (about 8 minutes per side).
3. Toss mixed greens with remaining olive oil and apple cider vinegar in a large bowl.
4. Top salad with sliced chicken and roasted vegetables. Serve warm.

Dietary Main Goals:
Muscle Building – Blood Sugar Management

Storage & Reheating:
Can be stored in an airtight container in the fridge for up to 2 days. Reheat in the oven or microwave.

Budget-Friendly Notes:
Chicken thighs are more cost-effective and flavorful than chicken breasts.
Serving Size: 1 plate

Nutrition Information: (Per Serving)
- Calories: 400 kcal
- Protein: 28g
- Carbohydrates: 20g
- Fiber: 6g
- Sugars: 5g
- Fat: 24g

34. Shrimp and Mango Lettuce Wraps

Yield: 1 serving   Prep Time: 10 minutes   Cooking Time: 5 minutes   Total Time: 15 minutes
Difficulty Level: Easy

Description: A refreshing and light meal that pairs succulent shrimp with sweet mango and creamy avocado, all wrapped in crisp lettuce leaves. Perfect for a quick and healthy lunch or dinner.

Ingredients:
- 225g / ½ lb wild-caught shrimp, peeled and deveined
- 70g / ½ mango, diced
- 4 large lettuce leaves (romaine or butter lettuce)
- 60g / ½ avocado, sliced
- 15ml / 1 tablespoon coconut oil
- 15ml / 1 tablespoon lime juice
- Salt to taste

Instructions:
1. Heat coconut oil in a skillet over medium heat. Add shrimp and cook for 3-4 minutes until pink.
2. Remove shrimp from heat and toss with lime juice and salt.
3. Assemble wraps by layering shrimp, mango, and avocado in lettuce leaves.
4. Roll tightly and serve immediately.

Dietary Main Goals:
Weight Loss – Blood Sugar Management

Storage & Reheating:
Best served fresh. Store in the fridge for up to 12 hours if needed.

Budget-Friendly Notes:
Use frozen shrimp to save costs and keep on hand for a quick meal.
Serving Size: 1 wrap

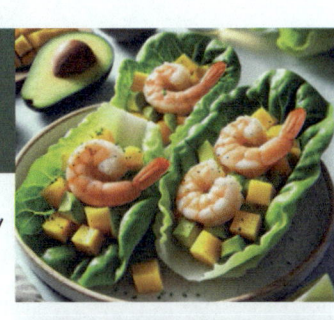

Nutrition Information: (Per Serving)
- Calories: 230 kcal
- Protein: 18g
- Carbohydrates: 12g
- Fiber: 4g
- Sugars: 6g
- Fat: 14g

35. Beef and Spinach Stuffed Acorn Squash

Yield: 1 serving Prep Time: 10 minutes Cooking Time: 35 minutes Total Time: 45 minutes
Difficulty Level: Moderate

Description: A hearty meal featuring roasted acorn squash stuffed with a flavorful ground beef and spinach mixture, perfect for a nourishing and filling dinner.

Ingredients:
- ½ acorn squash, halved and seeds removed
- 225g / ½ lb grass-fed ground beef
- 60g / 1 cup spinach, chopped
- 60g / ½ onion, diced
- 15ml / 1 tablespoon coconut oil
- 1g / ½ teaspoon dried thyme
- Salt and pepper to taste

Instructions:
1. Preheat oven to 375°F (190°C). Brush squash halves with coconut oil, season with salt and pepper, and bake for 30 minutes until tender.
2. While squash is baking, cook ground beef in a skillet over medium heat until browned.
3. Add onion, spinach, thyme, salt, and pepper to the skillet. Cook for 5 minutes until vegetables are soft.
4. Fill squash halves with the beef and spinach mixture and serve hot.

Dietary Main Goals:
Gut Health Support – Muscle Building

Storage & Reheating:
Can be refrigerated for up to 2 days. Reheat in the oven or microwave.

Budget-Friendly Notes:
Ground beef is a budget-friendly and versatile protein source.
Serving Size: 1 stuffed squash half

Nutrition Information: (Per Serving)
- Calories: 380 kcal
- Protein: 26g
- Carbohydrates: 20g
- Fiber: 4g
- Sugars: 4g
- Fat: 24g

---

36. Gut-Healing Turmeric Chicken Soup

Yield: 1 serving Prep Time: 10 minutes Cooking Time: 20 minutes Total Time: 30 minutes
Difficulty Level: Easy

Description: A soothing, anti-inflammatory soup made with turmeric, chicken, and nutrient-rich vegetables. This soup is perfect for supporting digestion and healing.

Ingredients:
- 240ml / 1 cup chicken bone broth
- 115g / 4 oz chicken breast, diced
- 30g / ¼ cup carrots, diced
- 30g / ¼ cup zucchini, diced
- 10g / 2 tablespoons leeks, sliced
- 5ml / 1 teaspoon coconut oil
- 1g / ¼ teaspoon ground turmeric
- Salt to taste

Instructions:
1. Heat the coconut oil in a small pot over medium heat. Add the sliced leeks and sauté for 3 minutes until soft.
2. Add the diced chicken, carrots, zucchini, and turmeric. Stir well and cook for 5 minutes until the chicken begins to brown.
3. Add the bone broth and bring to a boil. Lower the heat and simmer for 15 minutes.
4. Taste, season with salt, and serve hot.

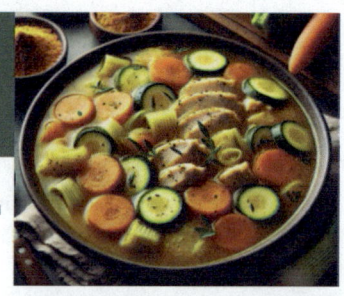

Dietary Main Goals:
Gut Health Support – Weight Loss

Storage & Reheating:
Store in the refrigerator for up to 2 days. Reheat on the stovetop or microwave.

Budget-Friendly Notes:
Use homemade bone broth to save on costs.
Serving Size: 1 bowl

Nutrition Information: (Per Serving)
- Calories: 210 kcal
- Protein: 22g
- Carbohydrates: 8g
- Fiber: 2g
- Sugars: 3g
- Fat: 10g

37. Herb-Roasted Lamb and Root Vegetables

- Yield: 1 serving
- Prep Time: 10 minutes
- Cooking Time: 35 minutes
- Total Time: 45 minutes
- Difficulty Level: Moderate

Description: A hearty meal featuring perfectly roasted lamb chops paired with tender root vegetables seasoned with fresh rosemary and garlic.

Ingredients:
- 225g / 1/2 lb pasture-raised lamb chops
- 120g / 1 cup carrots, diced
- 120g / 1 cup parsnips, diced
- 30ml / 2 tablespoons olive oil
- 5g / 1 tablespoon fresh rosemary, chopped
- 1g / 1 teaspoon garlic powder
- Salt and pepper to taste

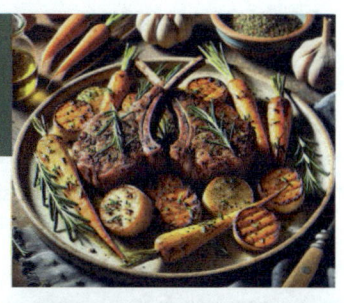

Instructions:
1. Preheat oven to 375°F (190°C). Toss carrots and parsnips in 1 tablespoon of olive oil, rosemary, garlic powder, salt, and pepper. Roast for 25 minutes.
2. Rub lamb chops with the remaining olive oil, salt, and pepper.
3. Sear the lamb in a skillet over medium heat for 3 minutes on each side, then transfer to the oven to finish cooking for 10 minutes.
4. Serve lamb with roasted root vegetables.

Dietary Main Goals:
Muscle Building – Blood Sugar Management

Storage & Reheating:
Best served fresh. Store in an airtight container in the fridge for up to 24 hours. Reheat in the oven.

Budget-Friendly Notes:
Opt for lamb cuts on sale or buy in bulk to reduce costs.
Serving Size: 1 plate

Nutrition Information: (Per Serving)
- Calories – 460 kcal
- Protein – 30g
- Carbohydrates – 18g
- Fiber – 4g
- Sugars – 5g
- Fat – 30g

---

38. Cauliflower Rice and Ginger Chicken Bowl

- Yield: 1 serving
- Prep Time: 10 minutes
- Cooking Time: 10 minutes
- Total Time: 20 minutes
- Difficulty Level: Easy

Description: A light and nourishing bowl featuring tender chicken, cauliflower rice, and broccoli, enhanced with the warm flavor of fresh ginger.

Ingredients:
- 225g / 1/2 lb chicken breast, diced
- 240g / 2 cups cauliflower rice
- 120g / 1 cup broccoli florets
- 30ml / 2 tablespoons coconut aminos
- 10g / 1 tablespoon fresh ginger, minced
- 15ml / 1 tablespoon coconut oil
- Salt to taste

Instructions:
1. Heat coconut oil in a skillet over medium heat. Cook the diced chicken with minced ginger for 5 minutes until browned.
2. Add cauliflower rice and broccoli, stirring to combine.
3. Pour in coconut aminos and cook for another 5 minutes.
4. Serve hot.

Dietary Main Goals:
Weight Loss – Gut Health Support

Storage & Reheating:
Can be stored in the fridge for up to 24 hours. Reheat in a skillet or microwave.

Budget-Friendly Notes:
Make your own cauliflower rice to save on costs.
Serving Size: 1 bowl

Nutrition Information: (Per Serving)
- Calories – 300 kcal
- Protein – 35g
- Carbohydrates – 10g
- Fiber – 3g
- Sugars – 2g
- Fat – 12g

39. Herb-Roasted Lamb and Root Vegetables

Yield: 1 serving Prep Time: 10 minutes Cooking Time: 20 minutes Total Time: 30 minutes
Difficulty Level: Moderate

Description: A nutritious and simple dish combining flavorful ground turkey with roasted spaghetti squash and tender mushrooms and spinach.

Ingredients:

- 225g / 1/2 lb ground turkey (pasture-raised)
- 240g / 1 cup roasted spaghetti squash, shredded
- 60g / 1/2 cup mushrooms, sliced
- 60g / 1/2 cup spinach, chopped
- 15ml / 1 tablespoon olive oil
- 1g / 1/2 teaspoon dried oregano
- Salt and pepper to taste

Instructions:

1. Cook ground turkey in a skillet over medium heat with olive oil, oregano, salt, and pepper for 8 minutes.
2. Add mushrooms and spinach to the skillet and cook for another 5 minutes until tender.
3. Serve turkey and vegetable mixture over roasted spaghetti squash.

Dietary Main Goals:
Muscle Building – Gut Health Support

Storage & Reheating:
Store in the refrigerator for up to 24 hours. Reheat in a skillet or microwave.

Budget-Friendly Notes:
Opt for bulk purchases of ground turkey to reduce overall costs.
Serving Size: 1 plate

Nutrition Information: (Per Serving)
- Calories – 320 kcal
- Protein – 30g
- Carbohydrates – 12g
- Fiber – 4g
- Sugars – 4g
- Fat – 18g

---

40. Seared Scallops with Garlic Spinach

Yield: 1 serving Prep Time: 5 minutes Cooking Time: 10 minutes Total Time: 15 minutes
Difficulty Level: Easy

Description: A delightful seafood dish with perfectly seared scallops served over garlicky sautéed spinach, finished with a fresh lemon drizzle.

Ingredients:

- 120g / 4 large sea scallops
- 120g / 2 cups fresh spinach
- 30ml / 2 tablespoons coconut oil
- 6g / 2 cloves garlic, minced
- 15ml / 1 tablespoon lemon juice
- Salt and pepper to taste

Instructions:

1. Heat 1 tablespoon of coconut oil in a skillet over medium-high heat. Sear scallops for 2 minutes on each side until golden.
2. In a separate skillet, heat the remaining coconut oil. Sauté garlic and spinach until wilted.
3. Serve scallops over spinach, drizzled with lemon juice.

Dietary Main Goals:
Muscle Building – Gut Health Support

Storage & Reheating:
Best served fresh. Scallops may lose their texture when reheated.

Budget-Friendly Notes:
Use frozen scallops to reduce costs.
Serving Size: 1 plate

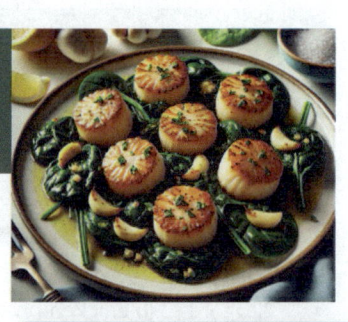

Nutrition Information: (Per Serving)
- Calories – 250 kcal
- Protein – 22g
- Carbohydrates – 6g
- Fiber – 2g
- Sugars – 1g
- Fat – 16g

41. Beef and Bok Choy Stir-Fry

Yield: 1 serving | Prep Time: 10 minutes | Cooking Time: 10 minutes | Total Time: 20 minutes
Difficulty Level: Easy

Description: A quick and healthy stir-fry featuring tender beef strips and bok choy, flavored with ginger and coconut aminos for a light and nutritious meal.

Ingredients:
- 115g / 4 oz grass-fed beef strips
- 240ml / 1 cup bok choy, chopped
- 30g / 2 tablespoons carrots, julienned
- 10ml / 2 teaspoons coconut aminos
- 5ml / 1 teaspoon coconut oil
- 1g / 1/4 teaspoon fresh ginger, minced
- Salt to taste

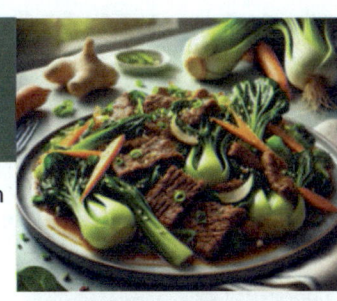

Instructions:
1. Prepare the ingredients: Chop the bok choy and julienne the carrots. Mince the ginger.
2. Heat the coconut oil in a skillet over medium-high heat.
3. Add beef strips and cook for 3-4 minutes until browned on all sides.
4. Stir-fry bok choy, carrots, and ginger. Add coconut aminos and salt.
5. Continue stir-frying for 4-5 minutes until vegetables are tender.
6. Serve hot.

Dietary Main Goals:
Weight Loss – Blood Sugar Management

Storage & Reheating:
Best served fresh but can be stored in an airtight container for up to 24 hours. Reheat in a skillet.

Budget-Friendly Notes:
Bok choy and beef strips are affordable ingredients, especially when bought in bulk.
Serving Size: 1 bowl

Nutrition Information: (Per Serving)
- Calories – 280 kcal
- Protein – 26g
- Carbohydrates – 10g
- Fiber – 3g
- Sugars – 4g
- Fat – 16g

---

42. Chicken and Artichoke Stew

Yield: 1 serving | Prep Time: 10 minutes | Cooking Time: 20 minutes | Total Time: 30 minutes
Difficulty Level: Moderate

Description: A warm and comforting stew with tender chicken and artichokes, rich in flavors and perfect for a cozy meal.

Ingredients:
- 115g / 4 oz chicken thighs, cubed
- 60ml / 1/4 cup artichoke hearts, chopped
- 30g / 1/4 cup carrots, diced
- 240ml / 1 cup chicken bone broth
- 5ml / 1 teaspoon olive oil
- 1g / 1/4 teaspoon dried thyme
- Salt and pepper to taste

Instructions:
1. Heat olive oil in a small pot over medium heat.
2. Add chicken and cook for 5 minutes until browned.
3. Stir in carrots, artichokes, thyme, salt, and pepper. Cook for 3-4 minutes.
4. Pour in bone broth, bring to a boil, and simmer for 10-12 minutes until vegetables are tender.
5. Serve hot.

Dietary Main Goals:
Gut Health Support – Weight Loss

Storage & Reheating:
Can be refrigerated for up to 2 days. Reheat on the stove or microwave.

Budget-Friendly Notes:
Using canned artichokes helps save money while adding a unique flavor to the stew.
Serving Size: 1 bowl

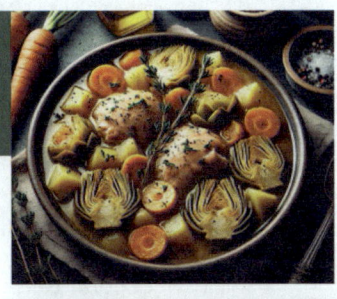

Nutrition Information: (Per Serving)
- Calories – 240 kcal
- Protein – 20g
- Carbohydrates – 10g
- Fiber – 3g
- Sugars – 2g
- Fat – 14g

43. AIP Turkey and Zucchini Skillet

Yield: 1 serving Prep Time: 10 minutes Cooking Time: 12 minutes Total Time: 22 minutes
Difficulty Level: Easy

Description: A quick and easy skillet meal combining ground turkey, zucchini, and carrots for a wholesome and satisfying dish.

Ingredients:
- 225g / 1/2 lb ground turkey
- 1 medium zucchini, diced
- 60g / 1/2 cup carrots, diced
- 30g / 1/4 onion, diced
- 30ml / 2 tablespoons coconut oil
- 1g / 1/4 teaspoon garlic powder
- Salt and pepper to taste
- Fresh parsley for garnish (optional)

Instructions:
1. Heat coconut oil in a skillet over medium heat.
2. Sauté onion for 2-3 minutes until softened.
3. Add ground turkey and cook until browned, about 5-7 minutes.
4. Stir in zucchini, carrots, garlic powder, salt, and pepper. Cook for 5 minutes until vegetables are tender.
5. Garnish with parsley and serve warm.

Dietary Main Goals:
Muscle Building - Blood Sugar Management

Storage & Reheating:
Can be stored in the fridge for up to 24 hours. Reheat in a skillet or microwave.

Budget-Friendly Notes:
Ground turkey is an affordable protein source, especially when bought in bulk.
Serving Size: 1 skillet

Nutrition Information: (Per Serving)
- Calories: 280 kcal
- Protein: 23g
- Carbohydrates: 8g
- Fiber: 2g
- Sugars: 4g
- Fat: 18g

44. AIP Salmon and Sweet Potato Salad

Yield: 1 serving Prep Time: 10 minutes Cooking Time: 25 minutes Total Time: 35 minutes
Difficulty Level: Easy

Description: This refreshing and nutrient-packed salad combines tender wild-caught salmon with roasted sweet potatoes and fresh mixed greens, finished with a light lemon dressing.

Ingredients:
- 1 salmon fillet (wild-caught, 4-6 oz / 115-170g)
- 1 small sweet potato, diced and roasted (150g)
- 2 cups mixed greens (120g)
- 1 tablespoon olive oil (15ml)
- 1 tablespoon lemon juice (15ml)
- Salt and pepper to taste
- Fresh herbs (dill or parsley) for garnish

Instructions:
1. Preheat the oven to 400°F (200°C). Toss diced sweet potatoes with 1 tablespoon of olive oil and roast for 20-25 minutes until tender.
2. While the sweet potatoes are roasting, cook the salmon fillet in a pan over medium heat for 3-4 minutes per side until cooked through.
3. In a bowl, combine the roasted sweet potatoes with mixed greens.
4. Drizzle with lemon juice and season with salt and pepper.
5. Place the cooked salmon on the salad, garnish with fresh herbs, and serve warm or chilled.

Dietary Main Goals:
Gut Health Support - Muscle Building

Storage & Reheating:
Best served fresh, but can be stored in an airtight container in the refrigerator for up to 24 hours. If chilled, enjoy cold or gently reheat the salmon.

Budget-Friendly Notes:
Using frozen salmon fillets can help reduce costs while still offering nutritional benefits.
Serving Size: 1 bowl

Nutrition Information: (Per Serving)
- Calories: 450 kcal
- Protein: 30g
- Carbohydrates: 30g
- Fiber: 5g
- Sugars: 8g
- Fat: 22g

CHAPTER 7: AIP DINNER RECIPES

45. One-Pot Chicken and Vegetable Stew

Yield: 4 servings Prep Time: 10 minutes Cooking Time: 25 minutes Total Time: 35 minutes
Difficulty Level: Easy

Description: A hearty and simple stew with tender chicken thighs and a medley of vegetables, perfect for a filling and nourishing dinner.

Ingredients:
- 1 lb chicken thighs, cubed (450g)
- 1 cup carrots, diced (120g)
- 1 cup celery, diced (100g)
- 1 cup sweet potatoes, diced (150g)
- 4 cups chicken bone broth (960ml)
- 1 tablespoon olive oil (15ml)
- 1 teaspoon dried thyme (1g)
- Salt and pepper to taste

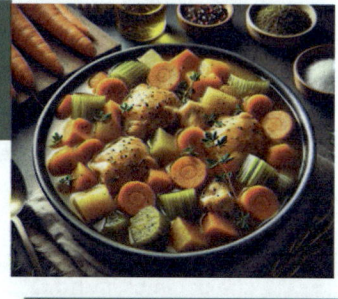

Nutrition Information: (Per Serving)
- Calories: 290 kcal
- Protein: 24g
- Carbohydrates: 18g
- Fiber: 4g
- Sugars: 4g
- Fat: 14g

Instructions:
1. Heat olive oil in a large pot over medium heat. Add cubed chicken thighs and cook until browned.
2. Add diced carrots, celery, and sweet potatoes. Cook for 5 minutes.
3. Pour in chicken bone broth and add thyme, salt, and pepper. Bring to a boil, then reduce heat and simmer for 20 minutes until the vegetables are tender.
4. Serve hot.

Dietary Main Goals:
Gut Health Support - Blood Sugar Management

Storage & Reheating:
Can be stored in the fridge for up to 3 days. Reheat on the stove or in the microwave.

Budget-Friendly Notes:
Using bone broth made from scratch or leftover chicken bones can help save on costs.
Serving Size: 1 bowl

46. AIP Shepherd's Pie with Cauliflower Mash

Yield: 4 servings Prep Time: 15 minutes Cooking Time: 30 minutes Total Time: 45 minutes
Difficulty Level: Moderate

Description: This paleo version of Shepherd's Pie features a flavorful ground lamb (or beef) base topped with creamy cauliflower mash, baked to golden perfection.

Ingredients:
- 1 lb ground lamb (or beef) (450g)
- 1 cup carrots, diced (120g)
- 1 cup zucchini, diced (120g)
- 1/2 onion, diced (75g)
- 2 cups cauliflower florets (300g)
- 2 tablespoons olive oil (30ml)
- 1 tablespoon coconut milk (15ml)
- 1/2 teaspoon garlic powder (1g)
- Salt and pepper to taste

Nutrition Information: (Per Serving)
- Calories: 360 kcal
- Protein: 30g
- Carbohydrates: 12g
- Fiber: 5g
- Sugars: 3g
- Fat: 22g

Instructions:
1. Preheat the oven to 375°F (190°C). Steam the cauliflower until tender, then blend it with coconut milk, garlic powder, salt, and pepper until smooth.
2. In a skillet, cook the ground lamb (or beef) with diced onion, carrots, and zucchini until browned.
3. Transfer the meat mixture to a baking dish and spread the cauliflower mash on top.
4. Bake for 20 minutes until golden.
5. Serve hot.

Dietary Main Goals:
Weight Loss - Blood Sugar Management

Storage & Reheating:
Can be refrigerated for up to 3 days and reheated in the oven or microwave.

Budget-Friendly Notes:
Using ground beef instead of lamb can help reduce the cost while maintaining flavor.
Serving Size: 1 plate

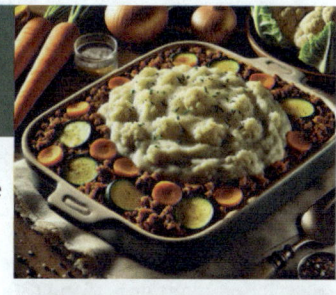

47. Roasted Garlic Herb Chicken with Root Vegetables

Yield: 4-6 servings   Prep Time: 15 minutes   Cooking Time: 70 minutes   Total Time: 85 minutes
Difficulty Level: Moderate

Description: A delicious, savory dish featuring a whole roasted chicken with aromatic garlic, rosemary, and hearty root vegetables like carrots and parsnips.

Ingredients:
- 1 whole chicken (3-4 lbs / 1.4-1.8 kg)
- 1 cup carrots, diced (150g)
- 1 cup parsnips, diced (150g)
- 1/2 cup onions, quartered (75g)
- 4 cloves garlic, minced (12g)
- 2 tablespoons olive oil (30ml)
- 1 tablespoon fresh rosemary, chopped (5g)
- Salt and pepper to taste

Nutrition Information: (Per Serving)
- Calories: 400 kcal
- Protein: 35g
- Carbohydrates: 10g
- Fiber: 3g
- Sugars: 2g
- Fat: 24g

Instructions:
1. Preheat the oven to 400°F (200°C). Rub the chicken with olive oil, minced garlic, chopped rosemary, salt, and pepper.
2. Place the chicken in a roasting pan and arrange the carrots, parsnips, and onions around it.
3. Roast the chicken for 60-70 minutes until the chicken reaches an internal temperature of 165°F (74°C) and the vegetables are tender.
4. Serve hot with the roasted vegetables.

Dietary Main Goals:
Muscle Building - Gut Health Support

Storage & Reheating:
Store leftovers in an airtight container in the fridge for up to 3 days. Reheat in the oven or microwave until warmed through.

Budget-Friendly Notes:
Whole chickens are more cost-effective than pre-cut pieces, providing more servings for your budget.
Serving Size: 1 plate

---

48. AIP Beef and Plantain Casserole

Yield: 4 servings   Prep Time: 10 minutes   Cooking Time: 25 minutes   Total Time: 35 minutes
Difficulty Level: Easy

Description: A comforting and hearty casserole that combines savory grass-fed beef, ripe plantains, and spinach, baked to golden perfection with coconut milk.

Ingredients:
- 1 lb ground beef (grass-fed, 450g)
- 2 ripe plantains, sliced (300g)
- 1 cup spinach, chopped (60g)
- 1/2 cup coconut milk (120ml)
- 1 tablespoon coconut oil (15ml)
- 1/2 teaspoon cinnamon (1g)
- Salt to taste

Nutrition Information: (Per Serving)
- Calories: 360 kcal
- Protein: 28g
- Carbohydrates: 25g
- Fiber: 4g
- Sugars: 8g
- Fat: 20g

Instructions:
1. Preheat the oven to 375°F (190°C). Cook the ground beef in a skillet until browned.
2. In a baking dish, layer half of the plantain slices, followed by the beef, spinach, and coconut milk. Top with the remaining plantain slices.
3. Bake for 25 minutes until the plantains are golden brown.
4. Serve hot.

Dietary Main Goals:
Gut Health Support - Blood Sugar Management

Storage & Reheating:
Store in the refrigerator for up to 3 days. Reheat in the oven or microwave until warmed.

Budget-Friendly Notes:
Plantains and ground beef are affordable staples, and using frozen spinach can reduce costs further.
Serving Size: 1 portion

49. Moroccan-Style Lamb Tagine

Yield: 4 servings Prep Time: 10 minutes Cooking Time: 60 minutes Total Time: 70 minutes
Difficulty Level: Moderate

Description: A warm, spiced Moroccan dish featuring tender lamb, butternut squash, and savory green olives, all simmered together with turmeric and ginger.

Ingredients:
- 1 lb lamb stew meat (450g)
- 1 cup butternut squash, diced (150g)
- 1/2 cup carrots, sliced (75g)
- 1/2 cup green olives (75g)
- 4 cloves garlic, minced (12g)
- 1 tablespoon olive oil (15ml)
- 1 teaspoon ground turmeric (2g)
- 1 teaspoon ground ginger (2g)
- Salt and pepper to taste

Instructions:
1. Heat olive oil in a large pot over medium heat. Add lamb and brown on all sides.
2. Add garlic, turmeric, ginger, salt, and pepper. Cook for 2 minutes until fragrant.
3. Add the butternut squash, carrots, and green olives. Cover with water and simmer for 1 hour until lamb is tender.
4. Serve hot.

Dietary Main Goals:
Weight Loss - Gut Health Support

Storage & Reheating:
Store in the refrigerator for up to 3 days. Reheat gently on the stove or microwave

Budget-Friendly Notes:
Lamb can be a more expensive protein, but using stew cuts helps reduce costs while maintaining flavor.
Serving Size: 1 bowl

Nutrition Information: (Per Serving)
- Calories: 420 kcal
- Protein: 30g
- Carbohydrates: 18g
- Fiber: 5g
- Sugars: 5g
- Fat: 26g

---

50. Italian-Inspired Stuffed Bell Peppers (AIP Version)

Yield: 4 servings Prep Time: 15 minutes Cooking Time: 30 minutes Total Time: 45 minutes
Difficulty Level: Moderate

Description: A healthy, flavorful AIP-compliant version of stuffed bell peppers filled with seasoned ground turkey, cauliflower rice, and mushrooms for a hearty meal.

Ingredients:
- 4 bell peppers (use non-nightshade substitutes like sweet peppers)
- 1 lb ground turkey (450g)
- 1 cup cauliflower rice (150g)
- 1/2 cup mushrooms, diced (75g)
- 1/2 onion, diced (75g)
- 2 tablespoons olive oil (30ml)
- 1 teaspoon dried basil (1g)
- Salt and pepper to taste

Instructions:
1. Preheat oven to 375°F (190°C). Sauté the diced onion and mushrooms in 1 tablespoon of olive oil until softened, about 5 minutes.
2. Add the ground turkey and cook until browned, breaking it apart as it cooks.
3. Stir in the cauliflower rice, basil, salt, and pepper. Cook for another 5 minutes.
4. Stuff the bell peppers with the turkey mixture and place them in a baking dish.
5. Bake for 30 minutes until the peppers are tender.
6. Serve hot.

Dietary Main Goals:
Weight Loss - Blood Sugar Management

Storage & Reheating:
Store leftovers in an airtight container in the fridge for up to 3 days. Reheat in the microwave or oven until warmed through.

Budget-Friendly Notes:
Ground turkey and cauliflower rice are affordable ingredients, and using non-nightshade substitutes for peppers can reduce costs.
Serving Size: 1 stuffed bell pepper

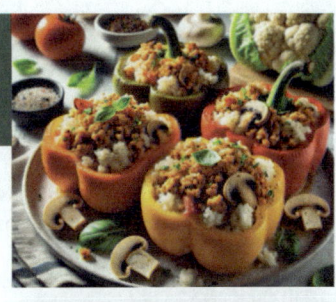

Nutrition Information: (Per Serving)
- Calories: 310 kcal
- Protein: 28g
- Carbohydrates: 14g
- Fiber: 4g
- Sugars: 6g
- Fat: 18g

51. Baked Cod with Lemon and Dill

Yield: 4-6 servings Prep Time: 5 minutes Cooking Time: 15 minutes Total Time: 20 minutes
Difficulty Level: Easy

Description: A light and fresh fish dish with cod fillets baked in a lemon and dill marinade for a simple, flavorful meal.

Ingredients:
- 4 cod fillets (wild-caught, 4-6 oz each)
- 2 tablespoons olive oil (30ml)
- 2 tablespoons lemon juice (30ml)
- 1 tablespoon fresh dill, chopped (5g)
- Salt and pepper to taste

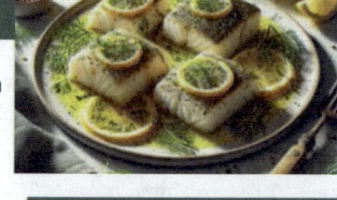

Instructions:
1. Preheat the oven to 375°F (190°C). Place cod fillets on a baking sheet lined with parchment paper.
2. Drizzle the fillets with olive oil and lemon juice, then sprinkle with dill, salt, and pepper.
3. Bake for 15 minutes, or until the cod is flaky and cooked through.
4. Serve hot.

Dietary Main Goals:
Muscle Building - Gut Health Support

Storage & Reheating:
Store in the fridge for up to 2 days. Reheat gently in the microwave or oven to avoid overcooking.

Budget-Friendly Notes:
Frozen cod fillets are often more affordable and work well for this recipe.
Serving Size: 1 cod fillet

Nutrition Information: (Per Serving)
- Calories: 200 kcal
- Protein: 28g
- Carbohydrates: 2g
- Fiber: 0g
- Sugars: 0g
- Fat: 10g

---

52. One-Pot Beef and Cabbage Skillet

Yield: 4 servings Prep Time: 10 minutes Cooking Time: 20 minutes Total Time: 30 minutes
Difficulty Level: Easy

Description: A simple and nutritious one-pot meal combining ground beef, cabbage, and carrots, with a touch of coconut aminos for flavor.

Ingredients:
- 1 lb ground beef (grass-fed, 450g)
- 4 cups green cabbage, shredded (400g)
- 1 cup carrots, shredded (150g)
- 1/2 onion, diced (75g)
- 2 tablespoons coconut aminos (30ml)
- 1 tablespoon olive oil (15ml)
- Salt and pepper to taste

Instructions:
1. Heat olive oil in a large skillet over medium heat. Add ground beef and cook until browned, about 5-7 minutes.
2. Add the onion, cabbage, and carrots to the skillet. Cook for 10 minutes until vegetables are tender.
3. Stir in the coconut aminos, salt, and pepper. Cook for another 5 minutes.
4. Serve hot.

Dietary Main Goals:
Weight Loss - Gut Health Support

Storage & Reheating:
Store in an airtight container in the fridge for up to 3 days. Reheat on the stovetop or microwave.

Budget-Friendly Notes:
Cabbage and carrots are inexpensive vegetables, making this a budget-friendly recipe.
Serving Size: 1 plate

Nutrition Information: (Per Serving)
- Calories: 290 kcal
- Protein: 24g
- Carbohydrates: 12g
- Fiber: 4g
- Sugars: 5g
- Fat: 16g

53. AIP Coconut Chicken Curry

Yield: 4 servings Prep Time: 10 minutes Cooking Time: 20 minutes Total Time: 30 minutes
Difficulty Level: Easy

Description: A rich and flavorful coconut chicken curry made with vibrant spices and vegetables. This AIP-friendly dish is both creamy and comforting.

Ingredients:
- 1 lb chicken breast, cubed (450g)
- 1 cup coconut milk (240ml)
- 1 cup carrots, sliced (150g)
- 1/2 cup green beans, chopped (75g)
- 2 tablespoons coconut oil (30ml)
- 1 tablespoon fresh ginger, minced (15g)
- 1 teaspoon turmeric powder (2g)
- Salt to taste

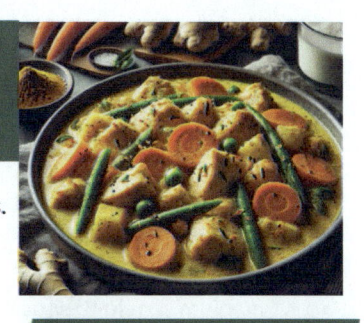

Nutrition Information: (Per Serving)
- Calories: 310 kcal
- Protein: 26g
- Carbohydrates: 12g
- Fiber: 3g
- Sugars: 4g
- Fat: 18g

Instructions:
1. Heat coconut oil in a large pan over medium heat. Add chicken and minced ginger, cooking until the chicken is browned, about 5 minutes.
2. Add carrots, green beans, turmeric, and salt. Cook for 5 minutes, stirring occasionally.
3. Pour in the coconut milk, bring to a simmer, and let it cook for 15 minutes until the vegetables are tender.
4. Serve hot with your favorite AIP-compliant sides.

Dietary Main Goals:
Gut Health Support - Weight Loss

Storage & Reheating:
Store leftovers in an airtight container in the fridge for up to 3 days. Reheat on the stovetop until heated through.

Budget-Friendly Notes:
Substitute fresh green beans for frozen if needed to save on costs.
Serving Size: 1 bowl of curry

54. AIP Beef and Broccoli Stir-Fry

Yield: 3 servings Prep Time: 10 minutes Cooking Time: 20 minutes Total Time: 20 minutes
Difficulty Level: Easy

Description: This quick and nutritious stir-fry combines tender beef, broccoli, and mushrooms for a satisfying, protein-packed meal.

Ingredients:
- 1 lb beef strips (grass-fed, 450g)
- 2 cups broccoli florets (300g)
- 1/2 cup mushrooms, sliced (75g)
- 1/4 cup coconut aminos (60ml)
- 2 tablespoons coconut oil (30ml)
- 1 tablespoon fresh ginger, grated (15g)
- Salt to taste

Nutrition Information: (Per Serving)
- Calories: 310 kcal
- Protein: 28g
- Carbohydrates: 14g
- Fiber: 4g
- Sugars: 6g
- Fat: 18g

Instructions:
1. Heat coconut oil in a skillet over medium-high heat. Add beef and cook until browned, about 5 minutes.
2. Add ginger, broccoli, mushrooms, and coconut aminos. Stir-fry for 5 minutes until the vegetables are tender.
3. Serve hot with your choice of AIP sides or cauliflower rice

Dietary Main Goals:
Muscle Building - Blood Sugar Management

Storage & Reheating:
Store in an airtight container in the fridge for up to 3 days. Reheat in a skillet or microwave until warm.

Budget-Friendly Notes:
Frozen broccoli can be used to cut costs.
Serving Size: 1 stir-fry portion

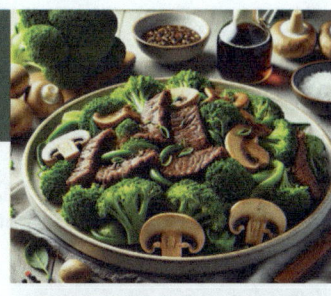

55. Spaghetti Squash with Turkey Meatballs

Yield: 4 servings Prep Time: 10 minutes Cooking Time: 30 minutes Total Time: 40 minutes
Difficulty Level: Moderate

Description: A delicious and healthy AIP-friendly twist on classic spaghetti and meatballs, using roasted spaghetti squash and tender turkey meatballs.

Ingredients:
- 1 medium spaghetti squash, halved and seeds removed (600g)
- 1 lb ground turkey (450g)
- 1/2 onion, diced (75g)
- 1/4 cup fresh basil, chopped (15g)
- 2 tablespoons olive oil (30ml)
- Salt and pepper to taste

Instructions:
1. Preheat the oven to 375°F (190°C). Place the spaghetti squash halves face down on a baking sheet and bake for 30 minutes.
2. While the squash is baking, mix ground turkey, diced onion, chopped basil, salt, and pepper, then form into meatballs.
3. Heat olive oil in a skillet and cook the turkey meatballs for about 10 minutes until browned and cooked through.
4. Once the squash is cooked, use a fork to scrape the squash into strands. Serve the squash topped with turkey meatballs.

Dietary Main Goals:
Weight Loss - Blood Sugar Management

Storage & Reheating:
Store spaghetti squash and meatballs separately in airtight containers in the fridge for up to 3 days. Reheat on the stovetop or microwave.

Budget-Friendly Notes:
Ground turkey and spaghetti squash are affordable, making this dish budget-friendly.
Serving Size: 1 bowl with meatballs and squash

Nutrition Information: (Per Serving)
- Calories: 340 kcal
- Protein: 30g
- Carbohydrates: 18g
- Fiber: 4g
- Sugars: 6g
- Fat: 18g

---

56. AIP-Friendly Chicken Fajitas

Yield: 4 servings Prep Time: 10 minutes Cooking Time: 15 minutes Total Time: 25 minutes
Difficulty Level: Easy

Description: A simple and delicious AIP-friendly fajita recipe using chicken breast, zucchini, and non-nightshade bell pepper substitutes, perfect for a flavorful and nutritious dinner.

Ingredients:
- 1 lb chicken breast, sliced (450g)
- 1 cup zucchini, sliced (150g)
- 1 cup bell pepper (non-nightshade substitute), sliced (150g)
- 1/2 onion, sliced (75g)
- 2 tablespoons olive oil (30ml)
- 1 tablespoon lemon juice (15ml)
- 1 teaspoon garlic powder (2g)
- Salt and pepper to taste

Instructions:
1. Heat olive oil in a large skillet over medium heat. Add sliced chicken and cook until browned, about 5 minutes.
2. Add zucchini, bell pepper, onion, lemon juice, garlic powder, salt, and pepper. Cook for another 10 minutes until the vegetables are tender and the chicken is fully cooked.
3. Serve hot, as-is or with AIP-compliant wraps.

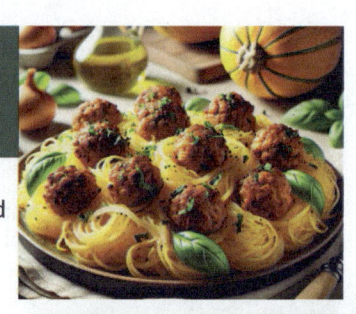

Dietary Main Goals:
Weight Loss - Gut Health Support

Storage & Reheating:
Store leftovers in an airtight container in the fridge for up to 3 days. Reheat in a skillet or microwave until warmed through.

Budget-Friendly Notes:
Zucchini and bell peppers are affordable and can be bought in bulk when in season for cost savings.
Serving Size: 1 portion of fajitas

Nutrition Information: (Per Serving)
- Calories: 280 kcal
- Protein: 26g
- Carbohydrates: 10g
- Fiber: 3g
- Sugars: 4g
- Fat: 16g

57. Baked Salmon with Dill and Asparagus

Yield: 4 servings | Prep Time: 5 minutes | Cooking Time: 20 minutes | Total Time: 25 minutes
Difficulty Level: Easy

Description: This baked salmon dish is a light and healthy meal, featuring fresh dill and asparagus for a perfect combination of flavors.

Ingredients:
- 4 salmon fillets (wild-caught, 115g each)
- 1 bunch asparagus, trimmed (200g)
- 2 tablespoons olive oil (30ml)
- 1 tablespoon lemon juice (15ml)
- 1 tablespoon fresh dill, chopped (5g)
- Salt and pepper to taste

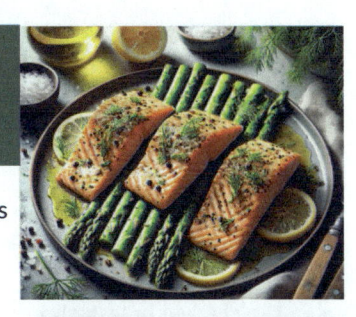

Instructions:
1. Preheat the oven to 375°F (190°C). Arrange salmon fillets and trimmed asparagus on a baking sheet.
2. Drizzle with olive oil and lemon juice, then sprinkle with dill, salt, and pepper.
3. Bake for 20 minutes or until the salmon is flaky and asparagus is tender.
4. Serve hot with a side of additional greens or salad if desired.

Dietary Main Goals:
Muscle Building - Gut Health Support

Storage & Reheating:
Store leftovers in an airtight container in the fridge for up to 2 days. Reheat in the oven at a low temperature or enjoy cold in a salad.

Budget-Friendly Notes:
Use frozen salmon fillets and asparagus to reduce costs while maintaining flavor and nutrition.
Serving Size: 1 fillet with asparagus

Nutrition Information: (Per Serving)
- Calories: 330 kcal
- Protein: 30g
- Carbohydrates: 6g
- Fiber: 3g
- Sugars: 2g
- Fat: 20g

---

58. AIP Braised Short Ribs with Garlic Cauliflower Mash

Yield: 4 servings | Prep Time: 15 minutes | Cooking Time: 2 hours | Total Time: 2 hours 15 minutes
Difficulty Level: Moderate

Description: A hearty AIP-friendly braised short rib recipe served with creamy garlic cauliflower mash, perfect for a cozy and satisfying dinner.

Ingredients:
- 2 lbs short ribs (grass-fed, 900g)
- 1 cup beef bone broth (240ml)
- 1/2 cup carrots, diced (75g)
- 4 cloves garlic, minced (12g)
- 1 tablespoon olive oil (15ml)
- 1 head cauliflower, steamed and mashed (500g)
- Salt and pepper to taste

Instructions:
1. Heat olive oil in a Dutch oven over medium heat. Sear short ribs on all sides until browned.
2. Add minced garlic and diced carrots, cooking for about 5 minutes.
3. Pour in bone broth, cover the pot, and let the ribs simmer for 2 hours until the meat is tender.
4. Meanwhile, steam cauliflower and mash with salt and pepper to serve alongside the ribs.
5. Serve the braised ribs over the garlic cauliflower mash.

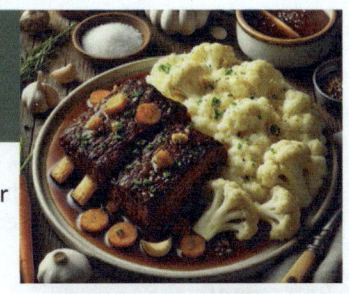

Dietary Main Goals:
Gut Health Support - Muscle Building

Storage & Reheating:
Store in an airtight container in the fridge for up to 3 days. Reheat in a covered pot over medium heat until warmed through.

Budget-Friendly Notes:
Opt for bone-in short ribs, which are more affordable and just as flavorful.
Serving Size: 1 portion of short ribs with mash

Nutrition Information: (Per Serving)
- Calories: 480 kcal
- Protein: 35g
- Carbohydrates: 12g
- Fiber: 4g
- Sugars: 3g
- Fat: 32g

59. Ginger Sesame Chicken Stir-Fry

Yield: 4 servings Prep Time: 10 minutes Cooking Time: 10 minutes Total Time: 20 minutes
Difficulty Level: Easy

Description: This quick stir-fry brings together ginger, sesame, and fresh vegetables for a light and savory meal that's easy to prepare.

Ingredients:
- 1 lb chicken breast, sliced (450g)
- 1 cup broccoli florets (150g)
- 1 cup bell pepper (non-nightshade), sliced (150g)
- 1/2 cup mushrooms, sliced (75g)
- 1/4 cup coconut aminos (60ml)
- 2 tablespoons coconut oil (30ml)
- 1 tablespoon fresh ginger, grated (15g)
- 1 tablespoon sesame seeds (15g)
- Salt to taste

Instructions:
1. Heat coconut oil in a skillet over medium heat. Add chicken slices and cook until browned, about 5 minutes.
2. Add ginger, broccoli, bell pepper, mushrooms, and coconut aminos. Stir-fry for another 5 minutes until the vegetables are tender.
3. Sprinkle with sesame seeds and serve hot with cauliflower rice or as-is.

Dietary Main Goals:
Muscle Building - Blood Sugar Management

Storage & Reheating:
Store leftovers in the fridge for up to 3 days. Reheat in a skillet with a little extra coconut oil.

Budget-Friendly Notes:
Swap fresh vegetables for frozen options to reduce costs.
Serving Size: 1 portion of chicken stir-fry

Nutrition Information: (Per Serving)
- Calories: 280 kcal
- Protein: 28g
- Carbohydrates: 8g
- Fiber: 3g
- Sugars: 2g
- Fat: 16g

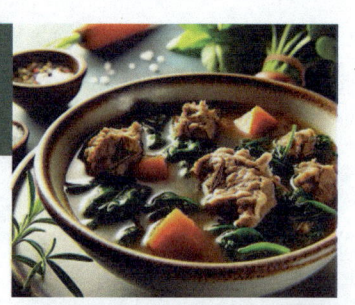

---

60. AIP-Friendly Chicken Fajitas

Yield: 4 servings Prep Time: 10 minutes Cooking Time: 15 minutes Total Time: 25 minutes
Difficulty Level: Moderate

Description: lamb meat with This hearty and nutritious lamb stew combines tender carrots, spinach, and a flavorful rosemary-infused broth. Perfect for a comforting dinner.

Ingredients:
- 1 lb lamb stew meat (450g)
- 2 cups spinach, chopped (60g)
- 1 cup carrots, diced (150g)
- 4 cups lamb bone broth (950ml)
- 1 tablespoon olive oil (15ml)
- 1 teaspoon dried rosemary (1g)
- Salt and pepper to taste

Instructions:
1. Heat olive oil in a pot over medium heat and brown the lamb stew meat.
2. Add diced carrots, rosemary, salt, and pepper. Cook for 5 minutes, stirring occasionally.
3. Pour in the lamb bone broth, bring to a boil, then reduce heat and simmer for 1 hour until the lamb is tender.
4. Add chopped spinach and cook for an additional 5 minutes until wilted.
5. Serve hot and enjoy.

Dietary Main Goals:
Gut Health Support - Muscle Building

Storage & Reheating:
Store in an airtight container in the fridge for up to 3 days. Reheat gently on the stovetop until warmed through.

Budget-Friendly Notes:
Use frozen spinach and pre-made bone broth to reduce costs while maintaining flavor.
Serving Size: 1 portion of stew

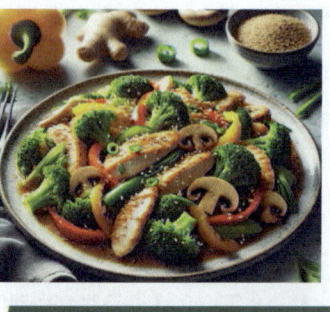

Nutrition Information: (Per Serving)
- Calories: 370 kcal
- Protein: 30g
- Carbohydrates: 10g
- Fiber: 3g
- Sugars: 3g
- Fat: 22g

61. Pork Tenderloin with Apple and Sage

Yield: 4 servings Prep Time: 5 minutes Cooking Time: 20 minutes Total Time: 25 minutes
Difficulty Level: Easy

Description: This baked salmon dish is a light and healthy meal, featuring fresh dill and asparagus for a perfect combination of flavors.

Ingredients:
- 1 lb pork tenderloin (450g)
- 2 apples, sliced (250g)
- 1/2 cup onions, sliced (75g)
- 1 tablespoon fresh sage, chopped (5g)
- 2 tablespoons olive oil (30ml)
- Salt and pepper to taste

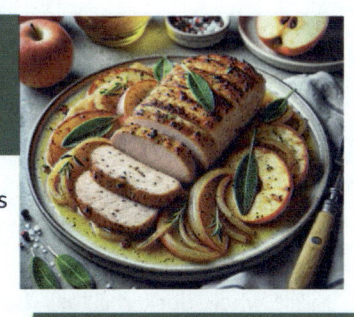

Instructions:
1. Preheat the oven to 375°F (190°C). Season the pork tenderloin with salt, pepper, and chopped sage.
2. Heat olive oil in a skillet over medium heat. Sear the pork on all sides until browned.
3. Add sliced apples and onions to the skillet, then transfer everything to the oven.
4. Roast for 25 minutes until the pork is cooked through and the apples are soft.
5. Serve hot with roasted apples and onions.

Dietary Main Goals:
Blood Sugar Management - Muscle Building

Storage & Reheating:
Store leftovers in an airtight container in the fridge for up to 3 days. Reheat in the oven at 350°F (175°C) until warmed through.

Budget-Friendly Notes:
Apples are affordable and can be swapped for pears if needed for a cost-effective meal.
Serving Size: 1 portion of pork tenderloin with apples

Nutrition Information: (Per Serving)
- Calories: 320 kcal
- Protein: 28g
- Carbohydrates: 14g
- Fiber: 3g
- Sugars: 8g
- Fat: 16g

62. AIP Shrimp and Cauliflower Fried Rice

Yield: 3 servings Prep Time: 10 minutes Cooking Time: 10 minutes Total Time: 20 minutes
Difficulty Level: Easy

Description: A light and flavorful AIP-friendly shrimp and cauliflower fried rice that's both easy to make and satisfying.

Ingredients:
- 1 lb shrimp, peeled and deveined (450g)
- 2 cups cauliflower rice (300g)
- 1/2 cup peas (optional) or zucchini (75g)
- 2 tablespoons coconut aminos (30ml)
- 1 tablespoon coconut oil (15ml)
- 1/2 teaspoon garlic powder (1g)
- Salt to taste

Instructions:
1. Heat coconut oil in a skillet over medium heat. Add shrimp and cook for 3-4 minutes until pink.
2. Add cauliflower rice, peas (or zucchini), coconut aminos, garlic powder, and salt. Stir-fry for 5 minutes until everything is heated through.
3. Serve hot as a main dish.

Dietary Main Goals:
Weight Loss - Gut Health Support

Storage & Reheating:
Store leftovers in the fridge for up to 2 days. Reheat in a skillet over medium heat until warmed through.

Budget-Friendly Notes:
Frozen shrimp and cauliflower rice can help reduce costs and make this dish more affordable.
Serving Size: 1 portion of shrimp fried rice

Nutrition Information: (Per Serving)
- Calories: 230 kcal
- Protein: 24g
- Carbohydrates: 8g
- Fiber: 2g
- Sugars: 3g
- Fat: 10g

63. Roasted Duck with Orange Glaze

Yield: 4-6 servings Prep Time: 10 minutes Cooking Time: 2 hours Total Time: 2 hours 10 minutes
Difficulty Level: Moderate

Description: A beautifully roasted duck brushed with a sweet and tangy orange glaze, perfect for special occasions or a comforting meal.

Ingredients:
- 1 whole duck (4-5 lbs / 1.8-2.3 kg)
- 1/2 cup orange juice (120 ml)
- 2 tablespoons honey (optional, 30 ml)
- 1 tablespoon fresh thyme, chopped (5 g)
- Salt and pepper to taste

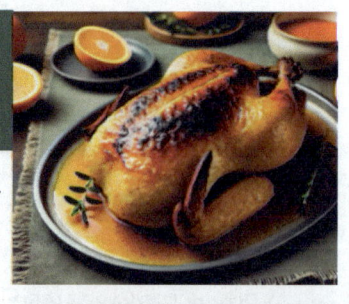

Instructions:
1. Preheat oven to 375°F (190°C). Season the duck with salt, pepper, and fresh thyme.
2. Roast the duck for 1.5 hours until the skin is golden and crisp.
3. Mix the orange juice and honey (if using) and brush over the duck. Roast for an additional 30 minutes, basting halfway through.
4. Serve hot, carving the duck and drizzling with any remaining orange glaze.

Dietary Main Goals:
Muscle Building - Gut Health Support

Storage & Reheating:
Store leftovers in an airtight container in the fridge for up to 3 days. Reheat in the oven at 350°F (175°C) until warm.

Budget-Friendly Notes:
Using seasonal or local oranges can reduce costs, and duck is often more affordable when bought whole.
Serving Size: 1 portion of roasted duck with glaze

Nutrition Information: (Per Serving)
- Calories: 480 kcal
- Protein: 35g
- Carbohydrates: 10g
- Fiber: 0g
- Sugars: 6g
- Fat: 34g

64. Greek-Style Chicken with Cauliflower Tabbouleh

Yield: 4 servings Prep Time: 15 minutes Cooking Time: 15 minutes Total Time: 30 minutes
Difficulty Level: Easy

Description: A light and fresh Mediterranean-inspired dish with grilled marinated chicken served over a flavorful cauliflower tabbouleh.

Ingredients:
- 1 lb chicken breast, cubed (450g)
- 2 cups cauliflower rice (300g)
- 1 cup cucumber, diced (150g)
- 1/2 cup fresh parsley, chopped (30g)
- 1/4 cup lemon juice (60ml)
- 3 tablespoons olive oil (45ml)
- Salt and pepper to taste

Instructions:
1. Marinate the chicken with lemon juice, olive oil, salt, and pepper for 30 minutes.
2. Grill the chicken until fully cooked, about 3-4 minutes per side.
3. In a bowl, combine cauliflower rice, diced cucumber, parsley, lemon juice, and olive oil. Mix well and season with salt and pepper.
4. Serve the grilled chicken over the cauliflower tabbouleh.

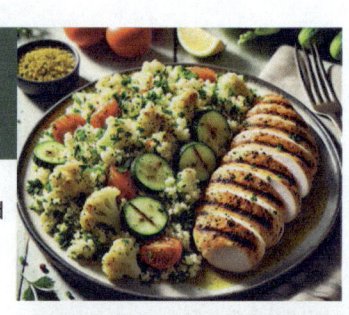

Dietary Main Goals:
Weight Loss - Blood Sugar Management

Storage & Reheating:
Store leftovers in the fridge for up to 2 days. Reheat the chicken on the stovetop and serve cold or room-temperature tabbouleh.

Budget-Friendly Notes:
Use frozen cauliflower rice for convenience, and chicken breast can be substituted with thighs for a more cost-effective option.
Serving Size: 1 portion of chicken and tabbouleh

Nutrition Information: (Per Serving)
- Calories: 280 kcal
- Protein: 30g
- Carbohydrates: 10g
- Fiber: 4g
- Sugars: 3g
- Fat: 12g

65. AIP Garlic-Infused Chicken Thighs with Roasted Vegetables

Yield: 1-2 servings Prep Time: 10 minutes Cooking Time: 30 minutes Total Time: 40 minutes
Difficulty Level: Easy

Description: Juicy garlic-infused chicken thighs paired with perfectly roasted Brussels sprouts and carrots for a simple yet flavorful AIP meal.

Ingredients:
- 2 bone-in, skin-on chicken thighs (about 300g)
- 1 tablespoon coconut oil (15ml)
- 1 teaspoon garlic powder (2g)
- 1/2 teaspoon dried thyme (1g)
- Salt and pepper to taste
- 1 cup Brussels sprouts, halved (150g)
- 1/2 cup carrots, chopped (75g)
- 1 tablespoon olive oil (15ml)

Instructions:
1. Preheat the oven to 400°F (200°C). Rub the chicken thighs with garlic powder, thyme, salt, and pepper.
2. Heat coconut oil in a skillet over medium heat. Sear the chicken thighs, skin side down, until golden, about 3-4 minutes.
3. Toss the Brussels sprouts and carrots with olive oil, salt, and pepper, then add them to the skillet with the chicken.
4. Transfer the skillet to the oven and roast for 25-30 minutes until the chicken reaches an internal temperature of 165°F (75°C).

Dietary Main Goals:
Gut Health Support - Muscle Building

Storage & Reheating:
Store in the fridge for up to 3 days. Reheat in the oven or on the stovetop for best results.

Budget-Friendly Notes:
Bone-in chicken thighs are often cheaper than boneless cuts, and seasonal root vegetables are more cost-effective.
Serving Size: 1 portion of chicken and vegetables

Nutrition Information: (Per Serving)
- Calories: 400 kcal
- Protein: 25g
- Carbohydrates: 20g
- Fiber: 6g
- Sugars: 4g
- Fat: 26g

66. AIP Beef and Butternut Squash

Yield: 1-2 servings Prep Time: 10 minutes Cooking Time: 35 minutes Total Time: 45 minutes
Difficulty Level: Easy

Description: A warming, hearty stew featuring grass-fed beef and nutrient-rich butternut squash, perfect for healing and satisfying hunger on the AIP diet.

Ingredients:
- 1/2 lb grass-fed beef stew meat, cubed (225g)
- 1 cup butternut squash, diced (150g)
- 1/2 cup carrots, diced (75g)
- 2 cups bone broth (beef or chicken, 480ml)
- 1 tablespoon coconut oil (15ml)
- 1/2 teaspoon ground turmeric (1g)
- 1/4 teaspoon ground ginger (0.5g)
- Salt to taste
- Fresh parsley for garnish (optional)

Instructions:
1. Heat the coconut oil in a large pot over medium heat. Add the beef stew meat and brown on all sides for about 5-7 minutes.
2. Add the diced butternut squash, carrots, turmeric, ginger, and a pinch of salt to the pot. Stir to combine and cook for 2 minutes.
3. Pour in the bone broth, bring the mixture to a boil, then reduce the heat to a simmer. Cover the pot and cook for 30-35 minutes until the beef is tender and the vegetables are cooked through.
4. Garnish with fresh parsley and serve hot.

Dietary Main Goals:
Gut Health Support - Muscle Building

Storage & Reheating:
Store leftovers in an airtight container in the fridge for up to 3 days. Reheat on the stovetop or microwave until warm.

Budget-Friendly Notes:
Substitute grass-fed beef with a more affordable cut of stew meat or bulk-bought butternut squash.
Serving Size: 1 portion of stew

Nutrition Information: (Per Serving)
- Calories: 350 kcal
- Protein: 25g
- Carbohydrates: 22g
- Fiber: 5g
- Sugars: 6g
- Fat: 18g

CHAPTER 8: AIP SNACKS AND SIDES RECIPESS

67. Gut-Healing Bone Broth

Yield: 8 cups | Prep Time: 10 minutes | Cooking Time: 12-24 hours | Total Time: 10 minutes
Difficulty Level: Easy

Description: A nutrient-rich bone broth made from grass-fed beef or chicken bones, perfect for gut healing and supporting overall health.

Ingredients:
- 2 lbs grass-fed beef bones or chicken bones (900g)
- 2 carrots, chopped (150g)
- 2 celery stalks, chopped (120g)
- 1 onion, quartered (100g)
- 4 cloves garlic, smashed
- 2 tablespoons apple cider vinegar (30ml)
- 10 cups water (2.4 liters)
- 1 teaspoon sea salt (5g)

Instructions:
1. Place all ingredients in a large pot or slow cooker.
2. Bring to a boil, then reduce heat to a low simmer and cook for 12-24 hours.
3. Strain the broth, discarding the solids. Store in glass jars or airtight containers.
4. Enjoy warm as a gut-healing drink or use in soups and stews.

Dietary Main Goals:
Gut Health Support - Weight Loss - Blood Sugar Management

Storage & Reheating:
Store in the fridge for up to 5 days or freeze for up to 3 months. Reheat on the stovetop or microwave before serving.

Budget-Friendly Notes:
Use leftover bones from roasts to create broth instead of buying bones separately.
Serving Size: 1 cup of bone broth

Nutrition Information: (Per Serving)
- Calories: 40 kcal
- Protein: 6g
- Carbohydrates: 2g
- Fiber: 0g
- Sugars: 1g
- Fat: 1g

---

68. Turmeric Ginger Healing Tea

Yield: 4 servings | Prep Time: 5 minutes | Cooking Time: 10 minutes | Total Time: 15 minutes
Difficulty Level: Easy

Description: A soothing, anti-inflammatory tea made from fresh turmeric and ginger, perfect for boosting immunity and reducing inflammation.

Ingredients:
- 1-inch fresh turmeric root, sliced (5g)
- 1-inch fresh ginger root, sliced (5g)
- 4 cups water (1 liter)
- 1 tablespoon honey (optional, 15ml)
- 1 tablespoon lemon juice (15ml)

Instructions:
1. Bring water, turmeric, and ginger to a boil in a pot.
2. Reduce heat and simmer for 10 minutes.
3. Strain the tea and stir in honey and lemon juice if desired.
4. Serve hot.

Dietary Main Goals:
Gut Health Support - Blood Sugar Management

Storage & Reheating:
Store in the fridge for up to 3 days. Reheat on the stovetop or microwave before serving.

Budget-Friendly Notes:
Fresh turmeric and ginger are affordable and widely available, making this a low-cost healing remedy.
Serving Size: 1 cup of healing tea

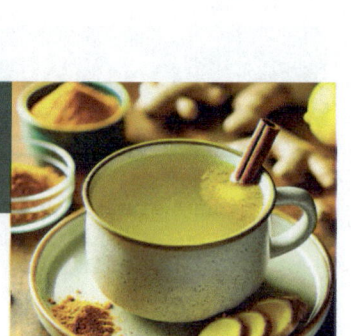

Nutrition Information: (Per Serving)
- Calories: 15 kcal
- Protein: 0g
- Carbohydrates: 4g
- Fiber: 0g
- Sugars: 3g
- Fat: 0g

69. Kale Chips with Sea Salt

Yield: 4 servings Prep Time: 5 minutes Cooking Time: 20 minutes Total Time: 25 minutes
Difficulty Level: Easy

Description: Crispy and delicious kale chips made with simple ingredients for a nutrient-dense, gut-friendly snack.

Ingredients:
- 4 cups kale leaves, stemmed and torn into pieces (120g)
- 2 tablespoons olive oil (30ml)
- 1/2 teaspoon sea salt (2.5g)

Instructions:
1. Preheat the oven to 300°F (150°C).
2. Toss the kale leaves with olive oil and sea salt.
3. Spread the kale on a baking sheet in a single layer.
4. Bake for 20 minutes, until crispy.
5. Cool and enjoy.

Dietary Main Goals:
Weight Loss - Gut Health Support

Storage & Reheating:
Store in an airtight container for up to 3 days at room temperature. No reheating required.

Budget-Friendly Notes:
Kale is an affordable, nutrient-packed leafy green, making this recipe a low-cost snack.
Serving Size: 1 cup of kale chips

Nutrition Information: (Per Serving)
- Calories: 70 kcal
- Protein: 2g
- Carbohydrates: 7g
- Fiber: 2g
- Sugars: 0g
- Fat: 5g

---

70. Sweet Potato Fries with Avocado Dip

Yield: 4 servings Prep Time: 10 minutes Cooking Time: 25 minutes Total Time: 35 minutes
Difficulty Level: Easy

Description: A satisfying side of baked sweet potato fries with a creamy avocado dip, perfect for snacking or a light meal.

Ingredients:
- 2 medium sweet potatoes, cut into fries (300g)
- 2 tablespoons olive oil (30ml)
- 1 teaspoon garlic powder (2g)
- 1/2 teaspoon sea salt (2.5g)
- 1 ripe avocado
- 1 tablespoon lime juice (15ml)

Instructions:
1. Preheat oven to 425°F (220°C).
2. Toss sweet potatoes with olive oil, garlic powder, and sea salt.
3. Arrange fries on a baking sheet in a single layer and bake for 25 minutes, turning once.
4. Mash the avocado with lime juice for a creamy dipping sauce.
5. Serve the fries with the avocado dip.

Dietary Main Goals:
Blood Sugar Management - Gut Health Support

Storage & Reheating:
Store fries and dip separately in airtight containers in the fridge for up to 2 days. Reheat fries in the oven at 350°F (180°C) until warm.

Budget-Friendly Notes:
Sweet potatoes are inexpensive and nutrient-rich, making this dish affordable.
Serving Size: 1 portion of fries with dip

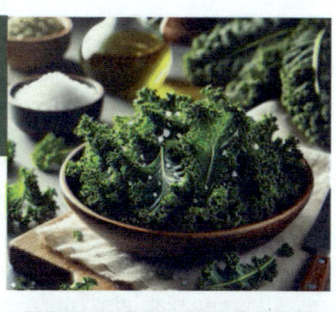

Nutrition Information: (Per Serving)
- Calories: 180 kcal
- Protein: 2g
- Carbohydrates: 22g
- Fiber: 5g
- Sugars: 4g
- Fat: 10g

71. AIP Plantain Chips

Yield: 4 servings Prep Time: 10 minutes Cooking Time: 20 minutes Total Time: 30 minutes
Difficulty Level: Easy

Description: Crispy plantain chips with a touch of sea salt, perfect for snacking or as a side dish.

Ingredients:
- 2 green plantains, thinly sliced (250g)
- 2 tablespoons coconut oil, melted (30ml)
- 1/2 teaspoon sea salt (2.5g)

Instructions:
1. Preheat the oven to 350°F (175°C).
2. Toss plantain slices with melted coconut oil and sea salt.
3. Arrange on a baking sheet in a single layer and bake for 20 minutes, until golden and crispy.
4. Cool and enjoy.

Dietary Main Goals:
Weight Loss - Blood Sugar Management

Storage & Reheating:
Store in an airtight container at room temperature for up to 3 days.

Budget-Friendly Notes:
Plantains are an affordable and versatile ingredient, making this snack budget-friendly.
Serving Size: 1 portion of plantain chips

Nutrition Information: (Per Serving)
- Calories: 130 kcal
- Protein: 1g
- Carbohydrates: 18g
- Fiber: 2g
- Sugars: 1g
- Fat: 6g

---

72. Zucchini Hummus

Yield: 2 cups Prep Time: 10 minutes Total Time: 35 minutes Difficulty Level: Easy

Description: A creamy, AIP-friendly alternative to traditional hummus, made from fresh zucchini and garlic for a light and flavorful dip.

Ingredients:
- 2 medium zucchinis, chopped (300g)
- 1/4 cup tahini (optional for non-strict AIP, 60ml)
- 2 tablespoons olive oil (30ml)
- 2 tablespoons lemon juice (30ml)
- 2 cloves garlic
- 1/2 teaspoon sea salt (2.5g)

Instructions:
1. Blend all ingredients in a blender or food processor until smooth.
2. Serve chilled with vegetable sticks or AIP-approved crackers.

Dietary Main Goals:
Gut Health Support - Blood Sugar Management

Storage & Reheating:
Store in the fridge for up to 3 days. No reheating required.

Budget-Friendly Notes:
Zucchini is widely available and inexpensive, making this a cost-effective recipe.
Serving Size: 1/4 cup of hummus

Nutrition Information: (Per Serving)
- Calories: 80 kcal
- Protein: 2g
- Carbohydrates: 6g
- Fiber: 1g
- Sugars: 2g
- Fat: 6g

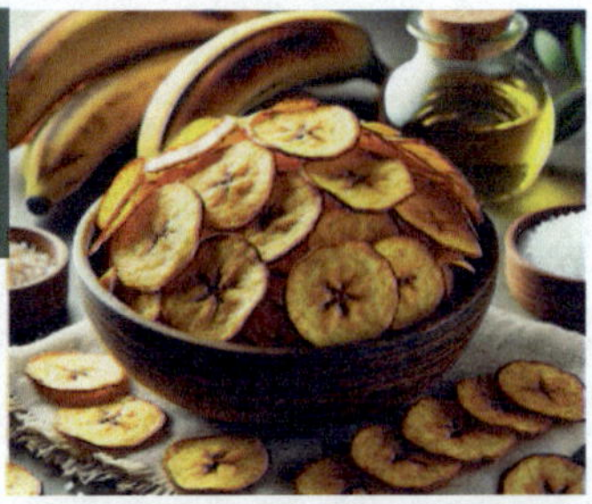

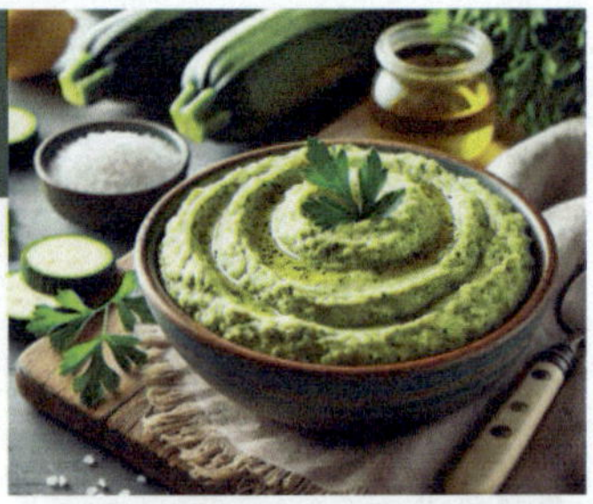

73. Cauliflower Rice Tabbouleh

Yield: 4 servings Prep Time: 10 minutes Total Time: 10 minutes Difficulty Level: Easy

Description: A fresh, grain-free tabbouleh made from cauliflower rice, cucumber, parsley, and lemon juice for a light and refreshing side dish.

Ingredients:
- 2 cups cauliflower rice (200g)
- 1/2 cup cucumber, diced (60g)
- 1/2 cup fresh parsley, chopped (30g)
- 1/4 cup red onion, finely diced (30g)
- 1/4 cup lemon juice (60ml)
- 2 tablespoons olive oil (30ml)
- Salt to taste

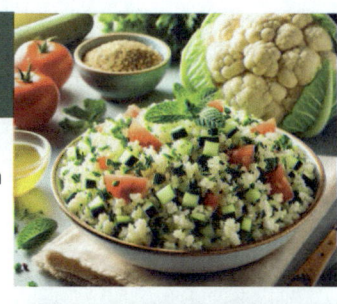

Instructions:
1. In a large bowl, combine all the ingredients and toss well.
2. Chill for 30 minutes before serving to allow the flavors to blend.

Dietary Main Goals:
Weight Loss - Gut Health Support

Storage & Reheating:
Store in an airtight container in the fridge for up to 3 days. No reheating required.

Budget-Friendly Notes:
Cauliflower and fresh herbs are affordable and can be found in most supermarkets.
Serving Size: 1 portion of cauliflower tabbouleh

Nutrition Information: (Per Serving)
- Calories: 70 kcal
- Protein: 2g
- Carbohydrates: 6g
- Fiber: 2g
- Sugars: 2g
- Fat: 5g

---

74. AIP Salsa Verde

Yield: 2 cups Prep Time: 10 minutes Total Time: 35 minutes Difficulty Level: Easy

Description: A fresh and zesty salsa verde perfect for pairing with AIP-approved chips or vegetable sticks.

Ingredients:
- 2 cups tomatillos, chopped (if tolerated, 240g)
- 1/2 cup cilantro, chopped (15g)
- 1/4 cup red onion, diced (40g)
- 2 tablespoons lime juice (30ml)
- 1 tablespoon olive oil (15ml)
- Salt to taste

Instructions:
1. Combine all ingredients in a bowl.
2. Chill for 30 minutes before serving with AIP chips or vegetable sticks.

Dietary Main Goals:
Gut Health Support - Weight Loss

Storage & Reheating:
Store in an airtight container in the fridge for up to 3 days. No reheating needed.

Budget-Friendly Notes:
Affordable and made with common fresh ingredients.
Serving Size: 1/4 cup salsa

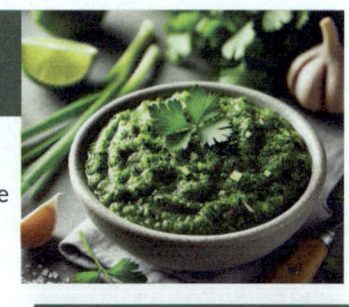

Nutrition Information: (Per Serving)
- Calories: 15 kcal
- Protein: 1g
- Carbohydrates: 3g
- Fiber: 1g
- Sugars: 1g
- Fat: 1g

75. Crispy Brussels Sprouts with Lemon

Yield: 4 servings Prep Time: 5 minutes Cooking Time: 25 minutes Total Time: 30 minutes
Difficulty Level: Easy

Description: Perfectly roasted Brussels sprouts with a zesty lemon kick, a savory and nutritious side dish.

Ingredients:
- 4 cups Brussels sprouts, halved (400g)
- 2 tablespoons olive oil (30ml)
- 1 tablespoon lemon juice (15ml)
- 1/2 teaspoon sea salt (2.5g)

Instructions:
1. Preheat oven to 400°F (200°C).
2. Toss Brussels sprouts with olive oil, lemon juice, and sea salt.
3. Spread on a baking sheet and roast for 25 minutes until crispy.
4. Serve warm.

Dietary Main Goals:
Gut Health Support - Blood Sugar Management

Storage & Reheating:
Store in an airtight container in the fridge for up to 3 days. Reheat in the oven at 350°F (175°C) for 5-10 minutes until warm.

Budget-Friendly Notes:
Brussels sprouts are affordable and readily available.
Serving Size: 1 cup of roasted Brussels sprouts

Nutrition Information: (Per Serving)
- Calories: 110 kcal
- Protein: 3g
- Carbohydrates: 10g
- Fiber: 4g
- Sugars: 2g
- Fat: 7g

---

76. Coconut-Date Energy Bites

Yield: 12 bites Prep Time: 10 minutes Total Time: 10 minutes Difficulty Level: Easy

Description: Sweet and satisfying AIP energy bites made with dates and coconut, perfect for a quick snack or post-workout treat.

Ingredients:
- 1 cup Medjool dates, pitted (200g)
- 1/2 cup shredded coconut (40g)
- 1 tablespoon coconut oil (15ml)
- 1/2 teaspoon cinnamon (1g)

Instructions:
1. Blend all ingredients in a food processor until a sticky dough forms.
2. Roll into small balls and refrigerate for 30 minutes.
3. Store in an airtight container.

Dietary Main Goals:
Gut Health Support - Weight Loss

Storage & Reheating:
Store in the fridge for up to a week. No reheating required.

Budget-Friendly Notes:
Dates and shredded coconut are cost-effective ingredients.
Serving Size: 1 bite

Nutrition Information: (Per Serving)
- Calories: 70 kcal
- Protein: 0g
- Carbohydrates: 11g
- Fiber: 1g
- Sugars: 9g
- Fat: 3g

77. Apple Cinnamon Chips

Yield: 4 servings | Prep Time: 10 minutes | Cooking Time: 2 hours | Total Time: 2 hours 10 minutes
Difficulty Level: Easy

Description: Light and crispy apple chips sprinkled with cinnamon, a sweet and healthy snack for any time of the day.

Ingredients:
- 2 large apples, thinly sliced (400g)
- 1 teaspoon cinnamon (2g)

Instructions:
1. Preheat the oven to 225°F (110°C).
2. Arrange apple slices on a baking sheet and sprinkle with cinnamon.
3. Bake for 2 hours until crisp.
4. Cool and enjoy.

Dietary Main Goals:
Blood Sugar Management - Weight Loss

Storage & Reheating:
Store in an airtight container at room temperature for up to 3 days. No reheating required.

Budget-Friendly Notes:
Apples and cinnamon are inexpensive and easy to find.
Serving Size: 1 portion of apple chips

Nutrition Information: (Per Serving)
- Calories: 50 kcal
- Protein: 0g
- Carbohydrates: 13g
- Fiber: 2g
- Sugars: 10g
- Fat: 0g

---

78. Carrot and Ginger Soup

Yield: 4 servings | Prep Time: 10 minutes | Cooking Time: 25 minutes | Total Time: 35 minutes
Difficulty Level: Easy

Description: A warming, nutrient-rich soup made from fresh carrots and ginger, perfect for a cozy meal or as a light appetizer.

Ingredients:
- 4 cups carrots, chopped (480g)
- 1-inch ginger root, sliced (10g)
- 4 cups bone broth (960ml)
- 1 tablespoon coconut oil (15ml)
- Salt to taste

Instructions:
1. Heat coconut oil in a pot over medium heat. Sauté carrots and ginger for 5 minutes.
2. Add bone broth and simmer for 20 minutes until carrots are soft.
3. Blend until smooth and serve warm.

Dietary Main Goals:
Gut Health Support - Weight Loss

Storage & Reheating:
Store in an airtight container in the fridge for up to 3 days. Reheat on the stove over low heat until warmed through.

Budget-Friendly Notes:
Carrots are inexpensive and bone broth can be made at home for a cost-effective meal.
Serving Size: 1 cup of soup

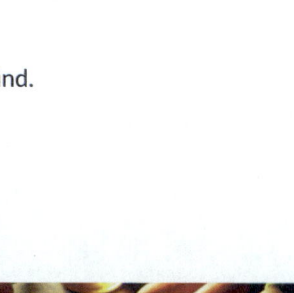

Nutrition Information: (Per Serving)
- Calories: 100 kcal
- Protein: 2g
- Carbohydrates: 16g
- Fiber: 4g
- Sugars: 8g
- Fat: 3g

79. Cucumber Dill Dip

Yield: 4 servings | Prep Time: 5 minutes | Total Time: 5 minutes | Difficulty Level: Easy

Description: A refreshing, creamy dip made with AIP-compliant coconut yogurt, perfect for pairing with vegetable sticks.

Ingredients:
- 1 cup coconut yogurt (AIP-compliant, 240ml)
- 1/2 cup cucumber, finely diced (75g)
- 1 tablespoon fresh dill, chopped (4g)
- 1 tablespoon lemon juice (15ml)
- Salt to taste

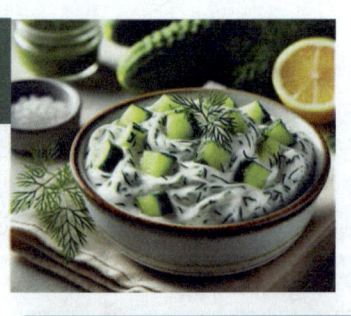

Instructions:
1. Mix all ingredients in a bowl.
2. Chill for 20 minutes before serving with vegetable sticks.

Dietary Main Goals:
Gut Health Support - Weight Loss

Storage & Reheating:
Store in an airtight container in the fridge for up to 3 days. No reheating required.

Budget-Friendly Notes:
This is a simple and cost-effective dip using basic ingredients.
Serving Size: 1/4 cup dip

Nutrition Information: (Per Serving)
- Calories: 45 kcal
- Protein: 1g
- Carbohydrates: 3g
- Fiber: 1g
- Sugars: 1g
- Fat: 3g

---

80. Coconut-Lemon Energy Balls

Yield: 12 balls | Prep Time: 10 minutes | Total Time: 10 minutes | Difficulty Level: Easy

Description: Sweet and tangy energy balls made from shredded coconut and lemon zest, perfect for a quick and healthy snack.

Ingredients:
- 1 cup shredded coconut (90g)
- 2 tablespoons coconut oil, melted (30ml)
- 1 tablespoon lemon zest (6g)
- 1 tablespoon honey (optional, 15ml)

Instructions:
1. Instructions:
2. Combine all ingredients in a bowl.
3. Roll into small balls and refrigerate for 30 minutes.
4. Store in an airtight container.

Dietary Main Goals:
Energy Boost - Gut Health Support

Storage & Reheating:
Store in the fridge for up to a week. No reheating required.

Budget-Friendly Notes:
These energy balls are made with affordable, pantry-friendly ingredients.
Serving Size: 1 energy ball

Nutrition Information: (Per Serving)
- Calories: 60 kcal
- Protein: 0g
- Carbohydrates: 4g
- Fiber: 1g
- Sugars: 3g
- Fat: 5g

81. Roasted Beet Chips

Yield: 4 servings | *Prep Time: 10 minutes* | *Cooking Time: 25 minutes* | *Total Time: 35 minutes*
Difficulty Level: Easy

Description: Crispy, homemade beet chips that are a perfect healthy alternative to traditional potato chips.

Ingredients:
- 3 medium beets, thinly sliced (300g)
- 2 tablespoons olive oil (30ml)
- 1/2 teaspoon sea salt (2.5g)

Instructions:
1. Preheat oven to 350°F (175°C).
2. Toss beet slices with olive oil and sea salt.
3. Arrange on a baking sheet and bake for 25-30 minutes until crispy.
4. Cool and enjoy.

Dietary Main Goals:
Blood Sugar Management - Weight Loss

Storage & Reheating:
Store in an airtight container at room temperature for up to 3 days. No reheating required.

Budget-Friendly Notes:
Beets are inexpensive and easy to find, making this a budget-friendly snack.
Serving Size: 1 portion of beet chips

Nutrition Information: (Per Serving)
- Calories: 80 kcal
- Protein: 2g
- Carbohydrates: 11g
- Fiber: 3g
- Sugars: 7g
- Fat: 4g

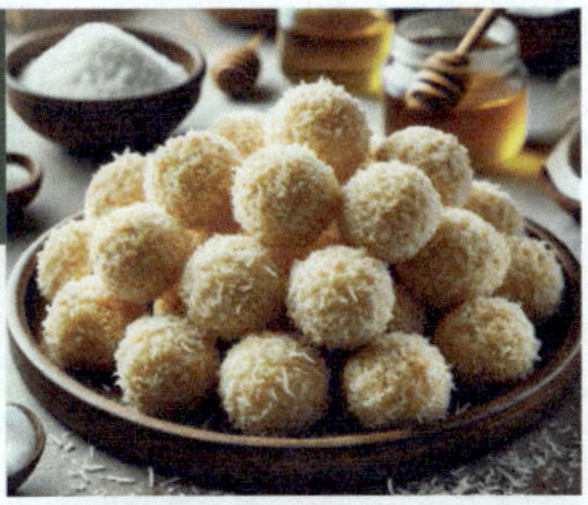

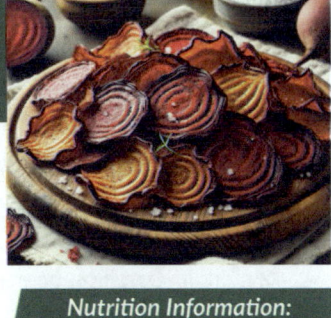

---

82. AIP Coconut Macaroons

Yield: 12 macaroons | *Prep Time: 10 minutes* | *Cooking Time: 15 minutes* | *Total Time: 25 minutes*
Difficulty Level: Easy

Description: These soft and chewy macaroons, made with coconut and naturally sweetened, are a perfect AIP-friendly treat.

Ingredients:
- 1 cup shredded coconut (90g)
- 2 tablespoons coconut flour (14g)
- 1/4 cup coconut oil, melted (60ml)
- 1 tablespoon honey (optional, 15ml)
- 1 teaspoon vanilla extract (AIP-compliant, 5ml)

Instructions:
1. Preheat oven to 350°F (175°C).
2. Mix all ingredients in a bowl until well combined.
3. Scoop small amounts onto a baking sheet lined with parchment paper.
4. Bake for 15 minutes until golden.
5. Cool and enjoy.

Dietary Main Goals:
Gut Health Support - Energy Boost

Storage & Reheating:
Store in an airtight container at room temperature for up to 3 days. No reheating required.

Budget-Friendly Notes:
With only a few ingredients, these macaroons are a cost-effective and delicious AIP dessert option.
Serving Size: 1 macaroon

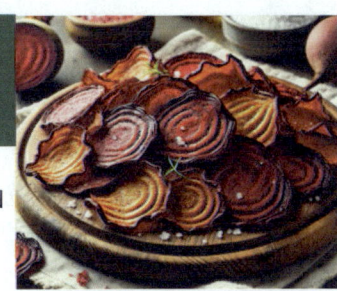

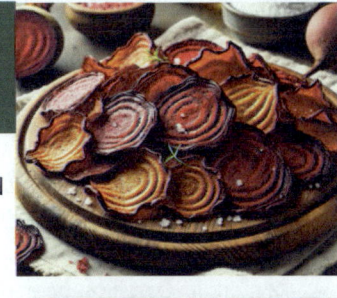

Nutrition Information: (Per Serving)
- Calories: 90 kcal
- Protein: 1g
- Carbohydrates: 6g
- Fiber: 1g
- Sugars: 4g
- Fat: 7g

83. AIP Baked Parsnip Fries

Yield: 2 servings | Prep Time: 10 minutes | Cooking Time: 25 minutes | Total Time: 35 minutes
Difficulty Level: Easy

Description: These crispy parsnip fries are a savory and nutrient-dense alternative to traditional fries, perfect as a side or snack.

Ingredients:
- 2 medium parsnips, peeled and cut into thin fries (200g)
- 1 tablespoon olive oil (15ml)
- 1/2 teaspoon garlic powder (2g)
- 1/4 teaspoon turmeric (1g)
- Salt to taste
- Fresh parsley for garnish (optional)

Instructions:
1. Preheat oven to 400°F (200°C).
2. Toss the parsnip fries in olive oil, garlic powder, turmeric, and salt.
3. Spread the fries in a single layer on a baking sheet lined with parchment paper.
4. Bake for 20-25 minutes, turning halfway through, until crispy and golden.
5. Remove from the oven, garnish with fresh parsley if desired, and serve warm.

Dietary Main Goals:
Weight Loss - Blood Sugar Management

Storage & Reheating:
Store in an airtight container in the fridge for up to 2 days. Reheat in the oven at 350°F (175°C) for 5-7 minutes until crispy.

Budget-Friendly Notes:
Parsnips are affordable and can easily replace more expensive root vegetables, making this a cost-effective side dish.
Serving Size: 1 portion of fries

Nutrition Information: (Per Serving)
- Calories: 150 kcal
- Protein: 2g
- Carbohydrates: 26g
- Fiber: 6g
- Sugars: 5g
- Fat: 5g

---

84. AIP Cucumber Avocado Salad

Yield: 1-2 servings | Prep Time: 5 minutes | Total Time: 5 minutes | Difficulty Level: Easy

Description: A refreshing and hydrating cucumber and avocado salad, tossed with fresh dill and a hint of lemon.

Ingredients:
- 1 cucumber, diced (200g)
- 1/2 avocado, diced (75g)
- 1 tablespoon olive oil (15ml)
- 1 tablespoon lemon juice (15ml)
- 1 tablespoon fresh dill, chopped (4g)
- Salt to taste

Instructions:
1. In a bowl, combine the diced cucumber and avocado.
2. Drizzle with olive oil and lemon juice.
3. Add the chopped dill and a pinch of salt. Toss everything gently to combine.
4. Serve chilled as a refreshing side dish or snack.

Dietary Main Goals:
Weight Loss - Gut Health Support

Storage & Reheating:
Store in the fridge for up to 1 day. Best served fresh and chilled.

Budget-Friendly Notes:
Avocados and cucumbers are usually inexpensive, and this recipe requires minimal ingredients, making it affordable and quick to prepare.
Serving Size: 1 portion of salad

Nutrition Information: (Per Serving)
- Calories: 180 kcal
- Protein: 2g
- Carbohydrates: 12g
- Fiber: 7g
- Sugars: 3g
- Fat: 16g

CHAPTER 9: AIP DESSERT AND BEVERAGE RECIPES

85. Apple Cinnamon Baked Apples

Yield: 4 servings | Prep Time: 10 minutes | Cooking Time: 30 minutes | Total Time: 40 minutes
Difficulty Level: Easy

Description: These soft and warm baked apples, enhanced with cinnamon and coconut, make for a comforting and AIP-friendly dessert.

Ingredients:
- 4 medium apples, cored (500g)
- 2 tablespoons coconut oil, melted (30ml)
- 1 tablespoon honey, optional (15ml)
- 1 teaspoon cinnamon (2.6g)
- 1/4 cup shredded coconut (20g)

Instructions:
1. Preheat oven to 350°F (175°C).
2. Place the cored apples in a baking dish. Drizzle with melted coconut oil and honey, then sprinkle with cinnamon and shredded coconut.
3. Bake for 25-30 minutes until the apples are soft.
4. Serve warm.

Dietary Main Goals:
Gut Health Support - Energy Boost

Storage & Reheating:
Store in an airtight container in the fridge for up to 2 days. Reheat in the oven at 350°F (175°C) for 5-7 minutes until warm.

Budget-Friendly Notes:
Apples are widely available and affordable, making this a cost-effective dessert option.
Serving Size: 1 baked apple

Nutrition Information: (Per Serving)
- Calories: 150 kcal
- Protein: 1g
- Carbohydrates: 27g
- Fiber: 5g
- Sugars: 20g
- Fat: 7g

---

86. Coconut Mango Sorbet

Yield: 4 servings | Prep Time: 5 minutes | Cooking Time: 2 hours | Total Time: 2 hours 5 minutes
Difficulty Level: Moderate

Description: A refreshing tropical sorbet made with mango, coconut milk, and a hint of lime, perfect for a light AIP-friendly dessert.

Ingredients:
- 2 cups mango chunks (fresh or frozen, 300g)
- 1/2 cup coconut milk (120ml)
- 1 tablespoon honey, optional (15ml)
- 1 tablespoon lime juice (15ml)

Instructions:
1. Blend all ingredients in a food processor until smooth.
2. Transfer to a container and freeze for 2 hours.
3. Scoop and serve.

Dietary Main Goals:
Gut Health Support - Energy Boost

Storage & Reheating:
Store sorbet in the freezer for up to 1 week. Allow to thaw for a few minutes before serving.

Budget-Friendly Notes:
Using frozen mango makes this dessert even more budget-friendly.
Serving Size: 1 serving of sorbet

Nutrition Information: (Per Serving)
- Calories: 120 kcal
- Protein: 1g
- Carbohydrates: 28g
- Fiber: 2g
- Sugars: 22g
- Fat: 4g

87. Blueberry Coconut Crumble

Yield: 4 servings Prep Time: 10 minutes Cooking Time: 20 minutes Total Time: 30 minutes
Difficulty Level: Easy

Description: A delicious and easy-to-make blueberry crumble with a coconut topping, perfect for a quick and healthy AIP dessert.

Ingredients:
- 2 cups fresh blueberries (300g)
- 1/2 cup shredded coconut (40g)
- 1/4 cup coconut flour (30g)
- 2 tablespoons coconut oil, melted (30ml)
- 1 tablespoon honey, optional (15ml)

Instructions:
1. Preheat oven to 350°F (175°C).
2. Place blueberries in a baking dish. In a separate bowl, mix shredded coconut, coconut flour, melted coconut oil, and honey.
3. Spread the crumble mixture over the blueberries.
4. Bake for 20 minutes until golden.
5. Serve warm.

Dietary Main Goals:
Gut Health Support - Blood Sugar Management

Storage & Reheating:
Store in an airtight container in the fridge for up to 2 days. Reheat in the oven at 350°F (175°C) for 5-7 minutes until warm.

Budget-Friendly Notes:
Blueberries are often available year-round, and this recipe uses minimal ingredients, making it affordable.
Serving Size: 1 portion of crumble

Nutrition Information: (Per Serving)
- Calories: 150 kcal
- Protein: 2g
- Carbohydrates: 24g
- Fiber: 5g
- Sugars: 16g
- Fat: 8g

88. Pineapple Coconut Popsicles

Yield: 6 popsicles Prep Time: 5 minutes Cooking Time: 4 hours Total Time: 4 hours 5 minutes
Difficulty Level: Moderate

Description: These tropical popsicles combine the sweetness of pineapple with the creaminess of coconut milk for a refreshing AIP-compliant treat.

Ingredients:
- 2 cups fresh pineapple, chopped (320g)
- 1 cup coconut milk (240ml)
- 1 tablespoon honey, optional (15ml)
- 1 teaspoon vanilla extract (AIP-compliant, 5ml)

Instructions:
1. Blend all ingredients until smooth.
2. Pour the mixture into popsicle molds and freeze for 4 hours.
3. Serve chilled.

Dietary Main Goals:
Gut Health Support - Energy Boost

Storage & Reheating:
Store in the freezer for up to 1 month.

Budget-Friendly Notes:
Fresh or frozen pineapple works equally well, allowing flexibility in cost.
Serving Size: 1 popsicle

Nutrition Information: (Per Serving)
- Calories: 70 kcal
- Protein: 1g
- Carbohydrates: 13g
- Fiber: 1g
- Sugars: 10g
- Fat: 3g

89. Peach and Coconut Milk Ice Cream

Yield: 4 servings Prep Time: 10 minutes Churning Time: 20 minutes Total Time: 1 hour 30 minutes
Difficulty Level: Moderate

Description: A dairy-free, AIP-friendly peach ice cream with a creamy coconut base and a hint of lemon.

Ingredients:
- 2 cups peaches, peeled and diced (300g)
- 1 cup coconut milk (240ml)
- 2 tablespoons honey, optional (30ml)
- 1 tablespoon lemon juice (15ml)

Nutrition Information: (Per Serving)
- Calories: 140 kcal
- Protein: 1g
- Carbohydrates: 26g
- Fiber: 2g
- Sugars: 22g
- Fat: 5g

Instructions:
1. Blend peaches, coconut milk, honey, and lemon juice until smooth.
2. Pour into an ice cream maker and churn according to the manufacturer's instructions.
3. Freeze for 1 hour before serving.

Dietary Main Goals:
Gut Health Support - Blood Sugar Management

Storage & Reheating:
Store in the freezer for up to 1 week.

Budget-Friendly Notes:
Use in-season peaches for a cost-effective option.
Serving Size: 1 serving of ice cream

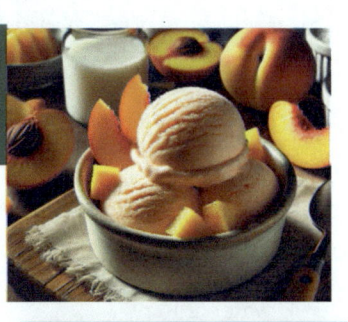

---

90. Coconut Banana Pudding

Yield: : 2 servings Prep Time: 5 minutes chilling Time: 1 hours Total Time: 1 hours 5 minutes
Difficulty Level: Easy

Description: A creamy, naturally sweet banana pudding with coconut milk, perfect for an AIP-friendly dessert or snack.

Ingredients:
- 2 ripe bananas, mashed (240g)
- 1/2 cup coconut milk (120ml)
- 1 tablespoon honey, optional (15ml)
- 1 teaspoon vanilla extract (AIP-compliant, 5ml)

Nutrition Information: (Per Serving)
- Calories: 140 kcal
- Protein: 1g
- Carbohydrates: 26g
- Fiber: 3g
- Sugars: 16g
- Fat: 5g

Instructions:
1. Blend all ingredients until smooth.
2. Chill in the refrigerator for 1 hour before serving.

Dietary Main Goals:
Gut Health Support - Energy Boost

Storage & Reheating:
Store in the fridge for up to 2 days.

Budget-Friendly Notes:
Bananas and coconut milk are affordable and accessible ingredients.
Serving Size: 1 serving of pudding

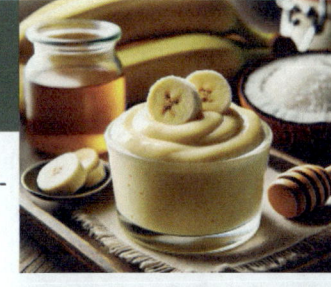

91. Apple Ginger Tea

Yield: 1 serving | Prep Time: 5 minutes | Cooking Time: 10 minutes | Total Time: 15 minutes
Difficulty Level: Easy

Description: A soothing and warming AIP tea with the flavors of fresh apple and ginger, perfect for a cozy beverage.

Ingredients:
- water (240ml)
- 1/4 tablespoon honey, optional (3.75ml)
- 1/4 apple, thinly sliced (45g)
- 1/4-inch ginger root, sliced (0.6cm)
- 1 cup

Instructions:
1. Bring water, apple slices, and ginger to a boil.
2. Simmer for 10 minutes.
3. Strain and add honey if desired. Serve hot.

Dietary Main Goals:
Gut Health Support – Anti-Inflammatory Benefits

Storage & Reheating:
Can be stored in the fridge for up to 2 days and reheated on the stove.

Budget-Friendly Notes:
Apples and ginger are inexpensive, making this an economical tea.
Serving Size: 1 cup of tea

Nutrition Information: (Per Serving)
- Calories: 20 kcal
- Protein: 0g
- Carbohydrates: 5g
- Fiber: 1g
- Sugars: 4g
- Fat: 0g

---

92. Berry Gelatin Cups

Yield: 1 serving | Prep Time: 10 minutes | Cook Time: 2 hours | Total Time: 2 hours 10 minutes
Difficulty Level: Easy

Description: These refreshing berry gelatin cups are perfect for a light, AIP-friendly dessert packed with antioxidants and flavor.

Ingredients:
- 1/2 cup mixed berries (blueberries, strawberries, 80g)
- 1/4 cup water (60ml)
- 1/4 tablespoon honey, optional (3.75ml)
- 1/4 tablespoon gelatin (3.75g)

Instructions:
1. Heat the water and honey until warm.
2. Sprinkle the gelatin into the warm water and stir until dissolved.
3. Divide the berries into a serving cup.
4. Pour the gelatin mixture over the berries and refrigerate for 2 hours until set.

Dietary Main Goals:
Gut Health Support – Anti-Inflammatory Benefits

Storage & Reheating:
Store in the fridge for up to 3 days. Not suitable for reheating.

Budget-Friendly Notes:
Fresh or frozen berries can be used depending on availability, keeping the cost low.
Serving Size: 1 gelatin cup

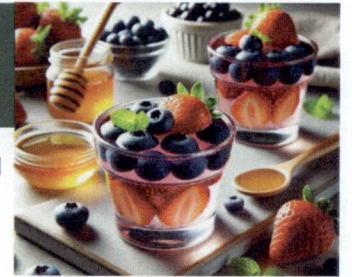

Nutrition Information: (Per Serving)
- Calories: 60 kcal
- Protein: 2g
- Carbohydrates: 12g
- Fiber: 3g
- Sugars: 8g
- Fat: 0g

93. AIP Carob Pudding

- Yield: 1 serving
- Prep Time: 5 minutes
- Cooking Time: 5 minutes
- Chilling Time: 10 minutes
- Total Time: 1 hour 10 minutes
- Difficulty Level: Easy

Description: A rich, creamy, chocolate-like pudding using AIP-compliant carob powder for a satisfying dessert without the need for chocolate.

Ingredients:
- 1/4 cup coconut milk (60ml)
- 2 tablespoons carob powder (15g)
- 1 tablespoon honey, optional (15ml)
- 1/2 tablespoon arrowroot starch (7.5g)

Instructions:
1. In a saucepan, whisk together all ingredients over medium heat until the mixture thickens.
2. Pour into a bowl and refrigerate for 1 hour before serving.

Dietary Main Goals:
Anti-Inflammatory Benefits – Energy Boost

Storage & Reheating:
Store in the fridge for up to 3 days. Not suitable for reheating.

Budget-Friendly Notes:
Carob powder and coconut milk are budget-friendly ingredients available in most stores.
Serving Size: 1 bowl of pudding

Nutrition Information: (Per Serving)
- Calories: 130 kcal
- Protein: 1g
- Carbohydrates: 24g
- Fiber: 3g
- Sugars: 16g
- Fat: 5g

94. Strawberry Coconut Milk Smoothie

- Yield: 1 serving
- Prep Time: 5 minutes
- Total Time: 5 minutes
- Difficulty Level: Easy

Description: A light and creamy strawberry smoothie made with coconut milk, perfect for a quick AIP-friendly snack or breakfast.

Ingredients:
- 1/2 cup strawberries (80g)
- 1/4 cup coconut milk (60ml)
- 2 tablespoons water (30ml)
- 1/4 tablespoon honey, optional (3.75ml)

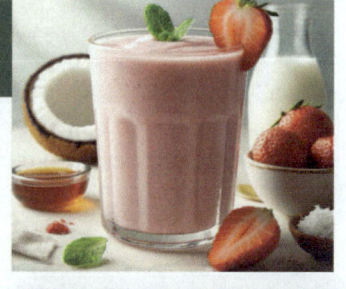

Instructions:
1. Blend all ingredients until smooth.
2. Serve chilled.

Dietary Main Goals:
Gut Health Support – Energy Boost

Storage & Reheating:
Best served fresh. Can be stored in the fridge for up to 1 day but may separate.

Budget-Friendly Notes:
Use fresh or frozen strawberries depending on availability to save on cost.
Serving Size: 1 glass of smoothie

Nutrition Information: (Per Serving)
- Calories: 90 kcal
- Protein: 1g
- Carbohydrates: 14g
- Fiber: 3g
- Sugars: 10g
- Fat: 4g

95. Lemon Ginger Bone Broth

Yield: 1 serving Prep Time: 5 minutes Churning Time: 10 minutes Total Time: 15 minutes
Difficulty Level: Easy

Description: A warm and soothing lemon ginger bone broth packed with nutrients and gut-healing properties.

Ingredients:
- 1 cup chicken bone broth (240ml)
- 1/4 tablespoon fresh ginger, sliced (3.75g)
- 1/2 tablespoon lemon juice (7.5ml)
- 1/4 tablespoon honey, optional (3.75ml)

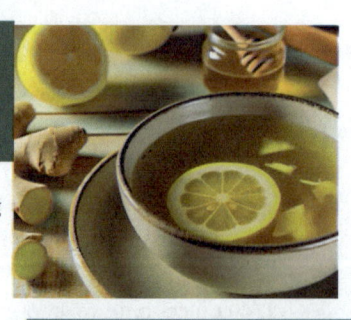

Instructions:
1. Heat bone broth with ginger over medium heat for 10 minutes.
2. Stir in lemon juice and honey if desired.
3. Serve hot.

Dietary Main Goals:
Gut Health Support – Immune System Boost

Storage & Reheating:
Can be stored in the fridge for up to 2 days and reheated on the stove.

Budget-Friendly Notes:
Homemade bone broth can reduce costs.
Serving Size: 1 cup of bone broth

Nutrition Information: (Per Serving)
- Calories: 30 kcal
- Protein: 6g
- Carbohydrates: 2g
- Fiber: 0g
- Sugars: 1g
- Fat: 0g

---

96. Coconut Berry Parfait

Yield: :1 serving Prep Time: 5 minutes Cooking Time: None Total Time:s 5 minutes Difficulty Level:Easy

Description: A creamy and refreshing parfait made with coconut yogurt and fresh berries, perfect for a single serving snack or dessert following the AIP diet.

Ingredients:
- 1/2 cup coconut yogurt (120g)
- 1/2 cup mixed berries (120g)
- 2 tablespoons shredded coconut (15g)

Instructions:
1. In a serving glass, layer the coconut yogurt, mixed berries, and shredded coconut.
2. Serve chilled.

Dietary Main Goals:
Gut Health Support

Storage & Reheating:
If needed, cover and refrigerate for up to 1 day.

Budget-Friendly Notes:
Using frozen mixed berries instead of fresh can reduce cost.
Serving Size: 1 parfait

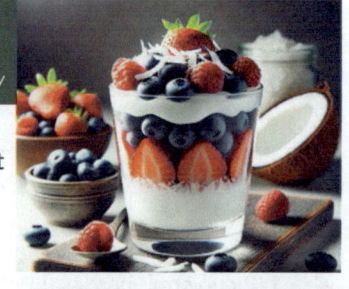

Nutrition Information: (Per Serving)
- Calories: 150
- Protein: 2g
- Carbohydrates: 16g
- Fiber: 4g
- Sugars: 10g
- Fat: 10g

97. Apple Cinnamon Coconut Cookies

Yield: 1 serving | Prep Time: 10 minutes | Churning Time: 15 minutes | Total Time: 25 minutes
Difficulty Level: Easy

Description: Chewy cookies with the flavors of apples, cinnamon, and coconut, ideal for an AIP-friendly treat for one.

Ingredients:
- 1/3 cup shredded coconut (40g)
- 1 tablespoon coconut flour (15g)
- 2 tablespoons applesauce (30g)
- 1 teaspoon honey, optional (5g)
- 1/8 teaspoon cinnamon (0.5g)

Instructions:
1. Preheat oven to 350°F (175°C).
2. Mix all ingredients together. Scoop small portions onto a baking sheet.
3. Bake for 15 minutes until golden. Let cool before enjoying.

Dietary Main Goals:
Gut Health Support

Storage & Reheating:
Store in an airtight container for up to 3 days.

Budget-Friendly Notes:
Applesauce can be made at home to save money.
Serving Size: 3 cookies

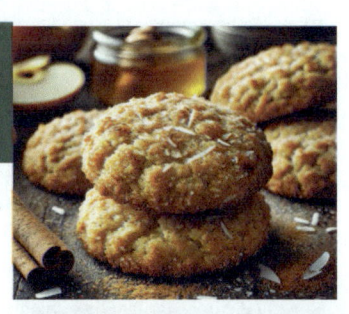

Nutrition Information: (Per Serving)
- Calories: 210
- Protein: 3g
- Carbohydrates: 16g
- Fiber: 6g
- Sugars: 8g
- Fat: 12g

---

98. Ginger Pear Herbal Tea

Yield: 1 serving | Prep Time: 5 minutes | Cooking Time: 10 minutes | Total Time: 5 minutes | Difficulty Level: Easy

Description: A soothing herbal tea made with ginger and pear for a warm, AIP-compliant drink.

Ingredients:
- 1/4 pear, thinly sliced (50g)
- 1-inch ginger root, sliced (2.5cm)
- cup water (240ml)
- 1/2 teaspoon honey, optional (2.5ml)

Instructions:
1. Bring water, pear slices, and ginger to a boil.
2. Simmer for 10 minutes. Strain and add honey if desired. Serve hot.

Dietary Main Goals:
Gut Health Support

Storage & Reheating:
Best served fresh. Can be refrigerated and reheated for up to 24 hours.

Budget-Friendly Notes:
Use leftover ginger and pears from other recipes.
Serving Size: 1 cup of tea

Nutrition Information: (Per Serving)
- Calories: 20
- Protein: 0g
- Carbohydrates: 5g
- Fiber: 1g
- Sugars: 3g
- Fat: 0g

99. Raspberry Coconut Milk Sorbet

Yield: 1 serving *Prep Time:* 5 minutes *Freezizing Time:* 2 hours *Total Time:* 2 hours 5 minutes
Difficulty Level: Easy

Description: A creamy and refreshing sorbet made with raspberries and coconut milk, ideal for a single-serving AIP dessert.

Ingredients:
- 1/2 cup raspberries, fresh or frozen (60g)
- 1/4 cup coconut milk (60ml)
- 1 teaspoon honey, optional (7.5ml)
- 1 teaspoon lemon juice (5ml)

Instructions:
1. Blend all ingredients until smooth.
2. Transfer to a container and freeze for 2 hours. Scoop and serve chilled.

Dietary Main Goals:
Gut Health Support – Weight Loss

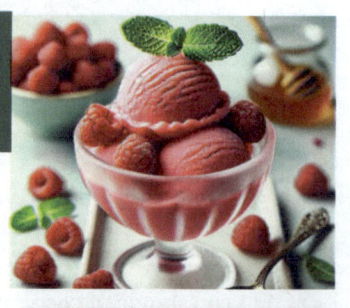

Storage & Reheating:
Store in a freezer-safe container for up to 1 week. Let thaw for a few minutes before serving.

Budget-Friendly Notes:
Use frozen raspberries to save on cost.
Serving Size: 1 sorbet serving

Nutrition Information: (Per Serving)
- Calories: 110
- Protein: 1g
- Carbohydrates: 20g
- Fiber: 6g
- Sugars: 12g
- Fat: 5g

100. Orange Cinnamon Hot Drink

Yield: :1 serving *Prep Time:* 5 minutes *Cooking Time:* 10 minutes *Total Time:s* 15 minutes *Difficulty Level:*Easy

Description: A warm, spiced drink made with orange and cinnamon for a cozy AIP-friendly treat.

Ingredients:
- 1 cup water (240ml)
- 2 orange slices (30g)
- 1 cinnamon stick
- 1 teaspoon honey, optional (5ml)

Instructions:
1. Bring water, orange slices, and cinnamon stick to a boil.
2. Simmer for 10 minutes. Strain and serve hot with honey if desired.

Dietary Main Goals:
Gut Health Support

Storage & Reheating:
Best consumed fresh. Can be reheated for up to 24 hours if stored in the fridge.

Budget-Friendly Notes:
Use oranges in season for cost-saving.
Serving Size: 1 cup of hot drink

Nutrition Information: (Per Serving)
- Calories: 30
- Protein: 0g
- Carbohydrates: 8g
- Fiber: 0g
- Sugars: 6g
- Fat: 0g

These AIP Dessert and Beverage Recipes satisfy sweet cravings and provide soothing, gut-friendly drinks while following the Paleo Autoimmune Protocol. Enjoy these delicious treats and beverages that are both healthy and AIP-compliant!

4-Week AIP Meal Plan

Day	Breakfast	Lunch	Snack	Dinner	Dessert	Beverage
Day 1	Apple Cinnamon Baked Apples	Sweet Potato Fries with Avocado Dip	Kale Chips with Sea Salt	One-Pot Chicken and Vegetable Stew	Coconut Mango Sorbet	Turmeric Ginger Healing Tea
Day 2	Coconut Banana Pudding	Beef and Broccoli Stir-Fry	AIP Plantain Chips	AIP Shepherd's Pie with Cauliflower Mash	Blueberry Coconut Crumble	Lemon Ginger Bone Broth
Day 3	Peach and Coconut Milk Ice Cream	Greek-Style Chicken with Cauliflower Tabbouleh	Zucchini Hummus with Vegetable Sticks	Roasted Garlic Herb Chicken with Root Vegetables	Berry Gelatin Cups	Apple Ginger Tea
Day 4	Strawberry Coconut Milk Smoothie	Cauliflower Rice Tabbouleh with Grilled Shrimp	Carrot and Ginger Soup	Moroccan-Style Lamb Tagine	Pineapple Coconut Popsicles	Orange Cinnamon Hot Drink
Day 5	Lemon Ginger Bone Broth	Beef and Plantain Casserole	Coconut-Date Energy Bites	Baked Cod with Lemon and Dill	Raspberry Coconut Milk Sorbet	Ginger Pear Herbal Tea
Day 6	Apple Cinnamon Baked Apples	One-Pot Beef and Cabbage Skillet	Roasted Beet Chips	Ginger Sesame Chicken Stir-Fry	AIP Carob Pudding	Turmeric Ginger Healing Tea
Day 7	Berry Gelatin Cups	Lamb and Spinach Stew	Coconut-Lemon Energy Balls	Spaghetti Squash with Turkey Meatballs	Coconut Berry Parfait	Apple Ginger Tea
Day 8	Strawberry Coconut Milk Smoothie	Shrimp and Cauliflower Fried Rice	Kale Chips with Sea Salt	AIP Shepherd's Pie with Cauliflower Mash	Apple Cinnamon Coconut Cookies	Lemon Ginger Bone Broth
Day 9	Coconut Banana Pudding	Roasted Garlic Herb Chicken with Root Vegetables	AIP Salsa Verde with Vegetable Sticks	Moroccan-Style Lamb Tagine	Pineapple Coconut Popsicles	Turmeric Ginger Healing Tea
Day 10	Blueberry Coconut Crumble	Baked Cod with Lemon and Dill	Carrot and Ginger Soup	One-Pot Chicken and Vegetable Stew	Coconut Mango Sorbet	Ginger Pear Herbal Tea
Day 11	Lemon Ginger Bone Broth	Greek-Style Chicken with Cauliflower Tabbouleh	Coconut-Lemon Energy Balls	Ginger Sesame Chicken Stir-Fry	Raspberry Coconut Milk Sorbet	Apple Ginger Tea
Day 12	Apple Cinnamon Baked Apples	One-Pot Beef and Cabbage Skillet	Roasted Beet Chips	Beef and Broccoli Stir-Fry	Coconut Berry Parfait	Orange Cinnamon Hot Drink
Day 13	Berry Gelatin Cups	Lamb and Spinach Stew	AIP Plantain Chips	Roasted Duck with Orange Glaze	AIP Carob Pudding	Apple Ginger Tea
Day 14	Peach and Coconut Milk Ice Cream	Beef and Plantain Casserole	Coconut-Date Energy Bites	Spaghetti Squash with Turkey Meatballs	Apple Cinnamon Coconut Cookies	Turmeric Ginger Healing Tea
Day 15	Strawberry Coconut Milk Smoothie	Greek-Style Chicken with Cauliflower Tabbouleh	Carrot and Ginger Soup	One-Pot Chicken and Vegetable Stew	Blueberry Coconut Crumble	Lemon Ginger Bone Broth
Day 16	Coconut Banana Pudding	Roasted Garlic Herb Chicken with Root Vegetables	Roasted Beet Chips	Moroccan-Style Lamb Tagine	Coconut Mango Sorbet	Ginger Pear Herbal Tea

Day 17	Apple Cinnamon Baked Apples	One-Pot Beef and Cabbage Skillet	Coconut-Lemon Energy Balls	Ginger Sesame Chicken Stir-Fry	Raspberry Coconut Milk Sorbet	Turmeric Ginger Healing Tea
Day 18	Berry Gelatin Cups	Beef and Broccoli Stir-Fry	AIP Salsa Verde with Vegetable Sticks	Lamb and Spinach Stew	AIP Carob Pudding	Apple Ginger Tea
Day 19	Peach and Coconut Milk Ice Cream	Shrimp and Cauliflower Fried Rice	AIP Plantain Chips	Spaghetti Squash with Turkey Meatballs	Apple Cinnamon Coconut Cookies	Orange Cinnamon Hot Drink
Day 20	Strawberry Coconut Milk Smoothie	Roasted Duck with Orange Glaze	Coconut-Date Energy Bites	Baked Cod with Lemon and Dill	Coconut Berry Parfait	Lemon Ginger Bone Broth
Day 21	Lemon Ginger Bone Broth	Greek-Style Chicken with Cauliflower Tabbouleh	Kale Chips with Sea Salt	One-Pot Chicken and Vegetable Stew	Blueberry Coconut Crumble	Apple Ginger Tea
Day 22	Coconut Banana Pudding	Beef and Plantain Casserole	Zucchini Hummus with Vegetable Sticks	Moroccan-Style Lamb Tagine	Pineapple Coconut Popsicles	Turmeric Ginger Healing Tea
Day 23	Apple Cinnamon Baked Apples	Baked Cod with Lemon and Dill	Roasted Beet Chips	Ginger Sesame Chicken Stir-Fry	Berry Gelatin Cups	Ginger Pear Herbal Tea
Day 24	Berry Gelatin Cups	One-Pot Beef and Cabbage Skillet	Coconut-Lemon Energy Balls	Beef and Broccoli Stir-Fry	Raspberry Coconut Milk Sorbet	Apple Ginger Tea
Day 25	Strawberry Coconut Milk Smoothie	Lamb and Spinach Stew	AIP Salsa Verde with Vegetable Sticks	Spaghetti Squash with Turkey Meatballs	Apple Cinnamon Coconut Cookies	Lemon Ginger Bone Broth
Day 26	Coconut Banana Pudding	Greek-Style Chicken with Cauliflower Tabbouleh	AIP Plantain Chips	Moroccan-Style Lamb Tagine	Coconut Berry Parfait	Orange Cinnamon Hot Drink
Day 27	Apple Cinnamon Baked Apples	Shrimp and Cauliflower Fried Rice	Roasted Beet Chips	Ginger Sesame Chicken Stir-Fry	AIP Carob Pudding	Turmeric Ginger Healing Tea
Day 28	Peach and Coconut Milk Ice Cream	Beef and Plantain Casserole	Coconut-Date Energy Bites	Baked Cod with Lemon and Dill	Raspberry Coconut Milk Sorbet	Apple Ginger Tea

The 4-Week AIP Meal Plan offers numerous benefits for individuals following the Paleo Autoimmune Protocol (AIP) diet, designed to reduce inflammation, support gut health, and promote overall wellness. This meal plan is tailored to help manage autoimmune conditions by eliminating common inflammatory foods and focusing on nutrient-dense, healing ingredients.

Benefits of the Meal Plan:

1. **Reduced Inflammation:** This plan minimizes potential triggers that can exacerbate autoimmune symptoms by avoiding inflammatory foods like grains, dairy, legumes, nuts, seeds, nightshades, and processed foods. Instead, it incorporates anti-inflammatory foods such as leafy greens, cruciferous vegetables, wild-caught fish, grass-fed meats, and healthy fats from coconut and olive oil.

2. **Gut Health Improvement:** Including bone broth, fermented vegetables, and fiber-rich produce promotes gut healing. Bone broth is rich in collagen, gelatin, and amino acids, which help repair the gut lining and reduce gut permeability. This is crucial for those with autoimmune disorders, as a healthy gut is the foundation of a strong immune system.

3. **Balanced Nutrition:** The plan ensures a balanced intake of macronutrients—proteins, healthy fats, and complex carbohydrates. Meals are rich in vitamins, minerals, and antioxidants, essential for supporting immune function, energy levels, and overall health.

4. **Stabilized Blood Sugar Levels:** This plan focuses on whole foods, lean proteins, and healthy fats, which can help stabilize blood sugar levels, reduce sugar cravings, and improve energy levels throughout the day.

Expected Outcomes:
Those who follow this meal plan can expect reduced autoimmune symptoms, improved digestion, increased energy levels, better mental clarity, and a greater sense of well-being. Eliminating potential irritants and including healing foods can help reset the immune system, allowing the body to heal and function optimally. With consistent adherence, individuals may also experience weight loss, reduced joint pain, and clearer skin.

Note:
This meal plan provides a balanced mix of breakfasts, lunches, snacks, dinners, desserts, and beverages for those following the AIP diet. You can adjust portions, ingredients, and recipes according to your needs and preferences.

Here is a Weekly Shopping List for the 4-week AIP Meal Plan. This list is organized by food categories, ensuring you have all the necessary ingredients to prepare the meals for each week.

Weekly Shopping List for the AIP Meal Plan

Week 1

Produce:
- Apples (8)
- Sweet potatoes (4)
- Kale (1 large bunch)
- Carrots (12)
- Celery (6 stalks)
- Onions (6)
- Garlic (2 bulbs)
- Zucchini (6)
- Bell peppers (non-nightshade substitute) (4)
- Spinach (1 large bag)
- Mixed berries (fresh or frozen, 4 cups)
- Mango (2 cups diced)
- Blueberries (2 cups)
- Avocado (4)
- Lemons (6)
- Limes (2)
- Oranges (4)
- Pears (4)
- Plantains (4)
- Ginger root (2-inch piece)
- Turmeric root (2-inch piece)
- Fresh herbs: cilantro, parsley, dill, rosemary, basil (1 bunch each)

Proteins:
- Chicken thighs (2 lbs)
- Chicken breasts (4 lbs)
- Ground beef (grass-fed, 2 lbs)
- Ground turkey (1 lb)
- Beef stew meat (2 lbs)
- Shrimp (2 lbs, wild-caught)
- Cod fillets (4)
- Salmon fillets (4)
- Lamb stew meat (2 lbs)
- Turkey meatballs (1 lb)
- Bone broth (8 cups, or make your own)

Healthy Fats:
- Olive oil (1 bottle)
- Coconut oil (1 jar)
- Avocado oil (1 bottle)

Pantry Staples:
- Coconut milk (6 cans)
- Coconut flour (1 bag)
- Coconut aminos (1 bottle)
- Coconut yogurt (AIP-compliant, 2 cups)
- Shredded coconut (1 bag)
- Honey (1 jar)
- Gelatin (1 box)
- Arrowroot starch (1 bag)
- Cinnamon (1 jar)
- Carob powder (1 bag)

Frozen:
- Frozen berries (optional, if fresh is not available) Spices & Seasonings:
- Sea salt
- Black pepper (if reintroduced)
- Garlic powder
- Dried thyme
- Dried basil
- Ground ginger
- Ground turmeric

Beverages:
- Herbal teas (ginger, turmeric, apple cinnamon, lemon ginger)
- Ingredients for bone broth (if making homemade)

Week 2

Produce:
- Apples (8)
- Sweet potatoes (4)
- Kale (1 large bunch)
- Carrots (12)
- Onions (6)
- Garlic (2 bulbs)
- Zucchini (6)
- Spinach (1 large bag)
- Mixed berries (fresh or frozen, 4 cups)
- Mango (2 cups diced)
- Blueberries (2 cups)
- Avocado (4)
- Lemons (6)
- Limes (2)
- Oranges (4)
- Pears (4)
- Plantains (4)
- Ginger root (2-inch piece)
- Fresh herbs: cilantro, parsley, dill, rosemary, basil (1 bunch each)

Proteins:
- Chicken thighs (2 lbs)
- Chicken breasts (4 lbs)
- Ground beef (grass-fed, 2 lbs)
- Lamb chops (1 lb)
- Salmon fillets (4)
- Ground turkey (1 lb)
- Shrimp (2 lbs, wild-caught)
- Duck (1 whole)
- Turkey meatballs (1 lb)
- Bone broth (8 cups, or make your own)

Healthy Fats:
- Olive oil (1 bottle)
- Coconut oil (1 jar)
- Avocado oil (1 bottle)
- Pantry Staples:
- Coconut milk (6 cans)
- Coconut flour (1 bag)
- Coconut aminos (1 bottle)
- Coconut yogurt (AIP-compliant, 2 cups)
- Shredded coconut (1 bag)
- Honey (1 jar)
- Gelatin (1 box)
- Arrowroot starch (1 bag)
- Cinnamon (1 jar)
- Carob powder (1 bag)

Frozen:
- Frozen berries (optional, if fresh is not available)
- Spices & Seasonings:
- Sea salt
- Black pepper (if reintroduced)
- Garlic powder
- Dried thyme
- Dried basil
- Ground ginger
- Ground turmeric

Beverages:
- Herbal teas (ginger, turmeric, apple cinnamon, lemon ginger)
- Ingredients for bone broth (if making homemade)

Week 3

Produce:
- Apples (8)
- Sweet potatoes (4)
- Kale (1 large bunch)
- Carrots (12)
- Celery (6 stalks)
- Onions (6)
- Garlic (2 bulbs)
- Zucchini (6)
- Bell peppers (non-nightshade substitute) (4)
- Spinach (1 large bag)
- Mixed berries (fresh or frozen, 4 cups)
- Mango (2 cups diced)
- Blueberries (2 cups)
- Avocado (4)
- Lemons (6)
- Limes (2)
- Oranges (4)
- Pears (4)
- Plantains (4)
- Ginger root (2-inch piece)
- Turmeric root (2-inch piece)
- Fresh herbs: cilantro, parsley, dill, rosemary, basil (1 bunch each)
- Cucumbers (2)
- Cauliflower (2 heads)
- Broccoli (2 heads)
- Asparagus (1 bunch)
- Butternut squash (1)

Proteins:
- Chicken thighs (2 lbs)
- Chicken breasts (4 lbs)
- Ground beef (grass-fed, 2 lbs)
- Ground turkey (1 lb)
- Beef stew meat (2 lbs)
- Shrimp (2 lbs, wild-caught)
- Cod fillets (4)
- Salmon fillets (4)
- Lamb stew meat (2 lbs)
- Turkey meatballs (1 lb)
- Duck (1 whole)
- Bone broth (8 cups, or make your own)

Healthy Fats:
- Olive oil (1 bottle)
- Coconut oil (1 jar)
- Avocado oil (1 bottle)

Pantry Staples:
- Coconut milk (6 cans)
- Coconut flour (1 bag)
- Coconut aminos (1 bottle)
- Coconut yogurt (AIP-compliant, 2 cups)
- Shredded coconut (1 bag)
- Honey (1 jar)
- Gelatin (1 box)
- Arrowroot starch (1 bag)
- Cinnamon (1 jar)
- Carob powder (1 bag)
- Apple cider vinegar (1 bottle)
- Bone broth ingredients (if making homemade)

Frozen:
- Frozen berries (optional, if fresh is not available)
- Spices & Seasonings:
- Sea salt
- Black pepper (if reintroduced)
- Garlic powder
- Dried thyme
- Dried basil
- Ground ginger
- Ground turmeric
- Dried rosemary
- Ground cinnamon
- Ground cloves

Beverages:
- Herbal teas (ginger, turmeric, apple cinnamon, lemon ginger)
- Ingredients for bone broth (if making homemade)

Week 4

Produce:
- Apples (8)
- Sweet potatoes (4)
- Kale (1 large bunch)
- Carrots (12)
- Celery (6 stalks)
- Onions (6)
- Garlic (2 bulbs)
- Zucchini (6)
- Bell peppers (non-nightshade substitute) (4)
- Spinach (1 large bag)
- Mixed berries (fresh or frozen, 4 cups)
- Mango (2 cups diced)
- Blueberries (2 cups)
- Avocado (4)
- Lemons (6)
- Limes (2)
- Oranges (4)
- Pears (4)
- Plantains (4)
- Ginger root (2-inch piece)
- Turmeric root (2-inch piece)
- Fresh herbs: cilantro, parsley, dill, rosemary, basil (1 bunch each)
- Cucumbers (2)
- Cauliflower (2 heads)
- Broccoli (2 heads)
- Asparagus (1 bunch)
- Butternut squash (1)

Proteins:
- Chicken thighs (2 lbs)
- Chicken breasts (4 lbs)
- Ground beef (grass-fed, 2 lbs)
- Ground turkey (1 lb)
- Beef stew meat (2 lbs)
- Shrimp (2 lbs, wild-caught)
- Cod fillets (4)
- Salmon fillets (4)
- Lamb stew meat (2 lbs)
- Turkey meatballs (1 lb)
- Duck (1 whole)
- Bone broth (8 cups, or make your own)

Healthy Fats:
- Olive oil (1 bottle)
- Coconut oil (1 jar)
- Avocado oil (1 bottle)
- Pantry Staples:
- Coconut milk (6 cans)
- Coconut flour (1 bag)
- Coconut aminos (1 bottle)
- Coconut yogurt (AIP-compliant, 2 cups)
- Shredded coconut (1 bag)
- Honey (1 jar)
- Gelatin (1 box)
- Arrowroot starch (1 bag)
- Cinnamon (1 jar)
- Carob powder (1 bag)
- Apple cider vinegar (1 bottle)
- Bone broth ingredients (if making homemade)
- Frozen:
- Frozen berries (optional, if fresh is not available)

Spices & Seasonings:
- Sea salt
- Black pepper (if reintroduced)
- Garlic powder
- Dried thyme
- Dried basil
- Ground ginger
- Ground turmeric
- Dried rosemary
- Ground cinnamon
- Ground cloves

Beverages:
- Herbal teas (ginger, turmeric, apple cinnamon, lemon ginger)
- Ingredients for bone broth (if making homemade)

By following this Weekly Shopping List, you will be well-prepared to make all the delicious and healing meals outlined in the 4-Week AIP Meal Plan, ensuring a continued focus on nutrient-dense. These anti-inflammatory foods support overall wellness and autoimmune management.

List of ingredients

Here is the detailed alphabetical list of ingredients, including the page numbers for each one:

A
Acorn Squash – Recipe 35 (Page 40)
Apple – Recipes 4, 9, 10, 16, 19, 22, 61, 77, 85, 91, 97 (Pages 24, 27, 28, 30, 32, 33, 53, 61, 65, 68, 71)
Apple Cinnamon – Recipes 10, 22, 85, 97 (Pages 27, 33, 65, 71)
Avocado – Recipes 6, 7, 23, 62, 79, 84 (Pages 25, 26, 34, 53, 62, 64)

B
Banana – Recipes 21, 90 (Pages 33, 67)
Beef – Recipes 24, 27, 31, 35, 41, 46, 48, 52, 54, 55, 58, 66 (Pages 34, 36, 38, 40, 43, 45, 46, 48, 49, 50, 51, 55)
Bell Peppers – Recipe 50 (Page 47)
Berries (Mixed) – Recipes 1, 6, 9, 92, 96 (Pages 23, 25, 27, 68, 70)
Blueberries – Recipes 9, 87 (Pages 27, 66)
Bone Broth – Recipes 26, 36, 67, 95 (Pages 35, 40, 56, 70)
Brussels Sprouts – Recipe 75 (Page 60)
Butternut Squash – Recipes 20, 28, 66 (Pages 32, 36, 55)

C
Carrot – Recipes 5, 11, 28, 78 (Pages 25, 28, 36, 61)
Cauliflower – Recipes 4, 12, 13, 19, 27, 31, 33, 38, 41, 46, 54, 58, 62, 64, 73 (Pages 24, 28, 29, 32, 36, 38, 39, 41, 43, 45, 49, 51, 53, 54, 59)
Chicken – Recipes 17, 23, 26, 28, 32, 33, 36, 42, 45, 47, 53, 56, 57, 59, 60, 65 (Pages 31, 34, 35, 36, 38, 39, 40, 43, 45, 46, 49, 50, 51, 52, 52, 55)
Cinnamon – Recipes 4, 9, 10, 16, 19, 22, 77, 85, 91, 95, 97, 100 (Pages 24, 27, 28, 30, 32, 33, 61, 65, 68, 70, 71, 72)
Coconut – Recipes 2, 6, 9, 14, 21, 87, 88, 89, 90, 92, 96, 97, 99 (Pages 23, 25, 27, 29, 33, 66, 66, 67, 67, 68, 70, 71, 72)
Collard Greens – Recipes 17, 23 (Pages 31, 34)
Cucumber – Recipes 79, 84 (Pages 62, 64)

D
Dates – Recipe 76 (Page 60)
Dill – Recipes 51, 57 (Pages 48, 51)

G
Ginger – Recipes 11, 28, 36, 78, 91, 95, 98 (Pages 28, 36, 40, 61, 68, 70, 71)
Ground Beef – Recipe 24 (Page 34)
Ground Turkey – Recipes 15, 43, 55 (Pages 30, 44, 50)

H
Herbs – Recipes 28, 37, 39, 47, 51, 57, 65 (Pages 36, 41, 42, 46, 48, 51, 55)

K
Kale – Recipes 7, 24, 69 (Pages 26, 34, 57)

L
Lamb – Recipes 37, 39, 49 (Pages 41, 42, 47)
Lemon – Recipes 30, 51, 57, 75, 95 (Pages 37, 48, 51, 60, 70)

M
Mango – Recipes 34, 86 (Pages 39, 65)

P
Parsnip – Recipe 83 (Page 64)
Peach – Recipe 89 (Page 67)
Pineapple – Recipes 88, 94 (Pages 66, 69)
Plantain – Recipes 8, 14, 48, 71 (Pages 26, 29, 46, 58)
Pumpkin – Recipe 18 (Page 31)

R
Raspberry – Recipe 99 (Page 72)

S
Salmon – Recipes 25, 30, 44, 51, 57 (Pages 35, 37, 44, 48, 51)
Sausage – Recipe 20 (Page 32)
Scallops – Recipe 40 (Page 42)
Sesame – Recipe 59 (Page 52)
Shrimp – Recipes 34, 62 (Pages 39, 53)
Spinach – Recipes 7, 12, 25, 32, 35, 38 (Pages 26, 28, 35, 38, 40, 41)
Squash – Recipes 15, 20, 28, 48, 50, 66 (Pages 30, 32, 36, 46, 47, 55)
Sweet Potato – Recipes 7, 19, 24, 31, 44, 66, 70 (Pages 26, 32, 34, 38, 44, 55, 57)

T
Turmeric – Recipes 29, 36, 67, 68, 95 (Pages 37, 40, 56, 56, 70)
Turkey – Recipes 15, 23, 43, 50, 55 (Pages 30, 34, 44, 47, 50)

Z
Zucchini – Recipes 15, 43, 62, 72 (Pages 30, 44, 53, 58)

This is the detailed alphabetical list of ingredients with their corresponding recipes and page numbers for the 100 listed recipes.

ABOUT ME

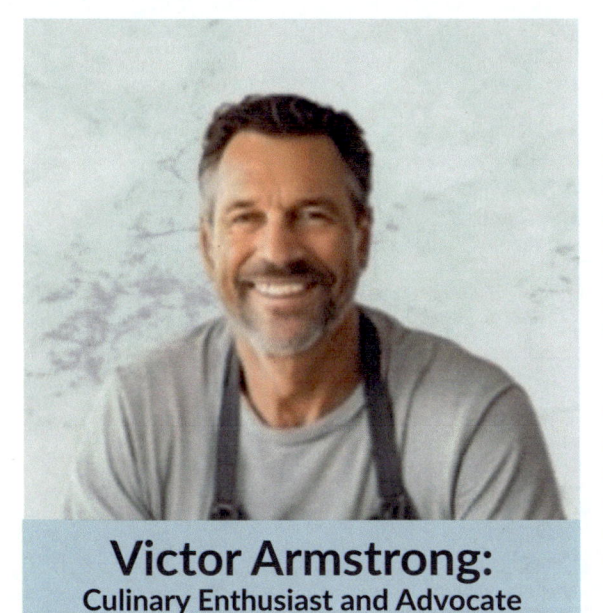

Victor Armstrong:
Culinary Enthusiast and Advocate for Transformative Eating

Victor Armstrong has always believed in the transformative power of food. His passion for cooking and helping others led him to author successful cookbooks that address specific health concerns. After his first book, "The Ultimate Paleo Autoimmune Protocol Cookbook for Beginners," became a hit, Victor turned his attention to another pressing issue—diabetes. His second cookbook, "The Ultimate Low Carb Recipe Book: High Protein Meal Prep, Diabetic-Friendly Diet Cookbook with Easy Low Carb Recipes," was released in 2025 to address the dietary needs of those managing diabetes and people seeking low-carb solutions for their health.

Victor's inspiration for this book came from personal experience—watching his own family struggle with blood sugar management. He knew firsthand the challenges of finding meals that were both satisfying and healthy. With a belief that food can heal and energize, Victor spent months in his kitchen developing recipes rich in protein, low in carbs, and full of bold flavors. His meals were designed to stabilize blood sugar, help manage weight, and maintain energy levels throughout the day.

Victor's cookbook stood out not just for its health benefits but for the joy it brought back to eating. His recipes weren't just functional; they were delicious, packed with vibrant flavors and textures. He made meal prep easy for busy individuals, offering simple, accessible instructions and a wide variety of cuisines. His book quickly gained popularity with diabetics and those on ketogenic diets, helping countless people embrace healthier lifestyles without sacrificing flavor.

Today, Victor's work continues to inspire readers to take control of their health one meal at a time, leaving a lasting impact on the world of healthy eating.

Made in United States
Troutdale, OR
01/20/2025